PRACTICAL PERIODONTAL PLASTIC SURGERY

PRACTICAL PERIODONTAL PLASTIC SURGERY

SECOND EDITION

Edited by

Serge Dibart, DMD
Professor and Chair
Graduate Program Director
Department of Periodontology and Oral Biology
Boston University School of Dental Medicine
Boston, MA, USA

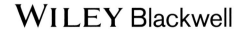

Library of Congress Cataloging-in-Publication Data

Names: Dibart, Serge, editor. | Preceded by (work): Dibart, Serge.
Practical periodontal plastic surgery.
Title: Practical periodontal plastic surgery / edited by Serge Dibart.
Description: Second edition. | Ames, Iowa : John Wiley & Sons
Inc., 2017. |
Preceded by: Practical periodontal plastic surgery / Serge Dibart,
Mamdouh
Karima. 1st ed. c2006. | Includes bibliographical references and
index.
Identifiers: LCCN 2016015697| ISBN 9781118360651 (cloth) |
ISBN 9781118985489
(Adobe PDF) | ISBN 9781118985502 (epub)
Subjects: | MESH: Periodontium–surgery | Reconstructive Surgical
Procedures–methods | Oral Surgical Procedures,
Preprosthetic–methods | Periodontics–methods
Classification: LCC RK361 | NLM WU 240 |
DDC 617.6/32059–dc23 LC record
available at https://lccn.loc.gov/2016015697

A catalogue record for this book is available from the British Library.

Set in 9.25/12pt HelveticaNeueLTStd by Aptara Inc., New Delhi,
India

Printed and bound in Singapore by Markono Print Media Pte Ltd

10 9 8 7 6 5 4 3 2 1

Contents

List of Contributors

James Belcher, DDS
Private practice limited to periodontics
Lakeland, FL, USA
Founder and head of the Periodontal Microsurgical
Institute, Lakeland, FL, USA

D.M. Diego Capri, DDS
Private practice limited to periodontics and dental implants
Bologna, Italy

Drew Czernick, DDS, MS
Private practice limited to periodontics and dental implants
Edmonton, Canada

Serge Dibart, DMD
Professor and Chair
Graduate Program Director
Department of Periodontology and Oral Biology
Boston University School of Dental Medicine
Boston, MA, USA

Thomas E. Van Dyke, DDS, PhD
Vice President for Clinical and Translational Research
Chair, Department of Applied Oral Sciences
Senior Member of the Staff
The Forsyth Institute, Boston, MA, USA

Ming Fang Su, DMD, MSc
Clinical Professor
Department of Periodontology and Oral Biology
Boston University School of Dental Medicine
Boston, MA, USA

Mamdouh Karima, BDS, CAGS, DSc
Assistant Professor of Periodontics
Clinical Director
Faculty of Dentistry
King Abdulaziz University
Jeddah, Saudi Arabia

Lorenzo Montesani, DDS
Private Practice
Rome, Italy

Luigi Montesani, MD, DMD
Private practice limited to periodontics, dental implants,
and prosthodontics
Rome, Italy

Yu-Chuan Pan, MD
Microsurgery Course Director
Department of Plastic Surgery
University of Texas M.D. Anderson Cancer Center
Houston, TX, USA

Ronaldo B. Santana DDS, MScD, DSc
Professor and Director
Graduate Program in Dentistry, Department of
Periodontology, Federal Fluminense
University, Dental School, Niteroi, Rio de Janeiro, Brazil

Bradford Towne, DMD
Clinical Assistant Professor
Department of Oral & Maxillofacial Surgery
Boston University Henry M. Goldman School of Dental
Medicine
Medical Director, OMS Ambulatory Care Operations
Boston Medical Center, Boston, MA

Foreword

Rarely does a scholarly work bridge the gap between academic underpinnings and utility for the practitioner. *Practical Periodontal Plastic Surgery* fulfills that role and is arguably the most useful book available on the subject today. Like all scholarly works, the content is not static and it requires updating. This second edition fills the gaps created by new discoveries and advances in the field since the publication of the first edition.

The essence of any practical guide to surgical procedures is the understanding of the biology, anatomy, and technical complexities of the procedures described. Omitting any of these elements limits the utility of the work. This book is indeed "practical" in every sense of the word. It is complete as well as directly useful. The clearly written chapters by the most expert educators and practitioners in the field provide an easily understood and valuable guide to experienced practitioners and students alike.

The discipline of periodontal plastic surgery has expanded exponentially in the past few years, making this second edition both timely and necessary. Life-long learning by the dental surgeon is the essence of successful, quality patient care. This book provides an excellent tool to manage the continued education needed for successful patient care by periodontists and others in our profession with an interest in the specialty. Our field is changing fast and everyone must keep abreast of innovations and changes to be successful caregivers in the 21st century.

In the spirit of scientific discovery and the development and implementation of those discoveries, this textbook, with new and expanded chapters, provides the scope and utility necessary for fostering expanded practical learning.

Thomas E. Van Dyke, DDS, PhD
Vice President for Clinical and Translational Research
Chair, Department of Applied Oral Sciences
Senior Member of the Staff
The Forsyth Institute

Chapter 1 Definition and Objectives of Periodontal Plastic Surgery

Serge Dibart, Mamdouh Karima, and Drew Czernick

Periodontal plastic surgery procedures are performed to prevent or correct anatomical, developmental, traumatic, or plaque disease-induced defects of the gingiva, alveolar mucosa, and bone (American Academy of Periodontology 1996).

THERAPEUTIC SUCCESS

This is the establishment of a pleasing appearance and form for all periodontal plastic procedures. Treatment of mucogingival deformities requires gingival augmentation procedures that address both a functional and esthetic component for the patient (American Academy of Periodontology 2015).

INDICATIONS

Gingival Augmentation

This is used to stop marginal tissue recession resulting from periodontal inflammation, toothbrush abrasion, or naturally occurring or orthodontically induced alveolar bone dehiscences. It facilitates plaque control around teeth or dental implants (Schrott et al. 2009; Lin et al. 2013) or in conjunction with the placement of fixed partial dentures (Nevins 1986; Jemt et al. 1994).

Root Coverage

The migration of the gingival margin below the cemento-enamel junction with exposure of the root surface is called *gingival recession*, which can affect all teeth surfaces, although it is most commonly found at the buccal surfaces (Murtomma et al. 1987). Gingival recession has been associated with tooth-brushing trauma, periodontal disease, tooth malposition, alveolar bone dehiscence, high muscle attachment, frenum pull, and iatrogenic dentistry (Wennstrom 1996). Gingival recessions can be classified in four categories based on the expected success rate for root coverage (Miller 1985):

- Class I: A recession not extending beyond the mucogingival line; normal interdental bone. Complete root coverage is expected.

- Class II: A recession extending beyond the mucogingival line; normal interdental bone. Complete root coverage is expected.

- Class III: A recession to or beyond the mucogingival line. There is a loss of interdental bone, with level coronal to gingival recession. Partial root coverage is expected.

- Class IV: A recession extending beyond the mucogingival line. There is a loss of interdental bone apical to the level of tissue recession. No root coverage is expected.

Root-coverage procedures are aimed at improving aesthetics, reducing root sensitivity, and managing root caries and abrasions.

Augmentation of the Edentulous Ridge

This is a correction of ridge deformities following tooth loss (facial trauma) or developmental defects (Allen et al. 1985; Hawkins et al. 1991). It is used in preparation for the placement of a fixed partial denture or implant-supported prosthesis when aesthetics and function could be otherwise compromised. Ridge deformities can be grouped into three classes (Seibert 1993):

- Class I: A horizontal loss of tissue with normal, vertical ridge height

- Class II: Vertical loss of ridge height with normal, horizontal ridge width

- Class III: Combination of horizontal and vertical tissue loss

Aberrant Frenulum

Frenectomy or frenotomy can be used to remove or apically reposition aberrant frenulum in order to close diastemas in conjunction with orthodontic therapy. It is used in treating gingival tissue recession aggravated by a frenum pull (Edwards 1977).

Prevention of Ridge Collapse Associated with Tooth Extraction (Socket Preservation)

The maintenance of socket space with a bone graft after extraction will help reduce the chances of alveolar ridge resorption and facilitate future implant placement.

Crown Lengthening

This is used when there is not enough dental tissue available (Yeh & Andreana 2004; Sharma et al. 2012) or to improve aesthetics (Bragger et al. 1992; Garber & Salama 1996; Sonick 1997).

Exposure of Nonerupted Teeth

The procedure is aimed at uncovering the clinical crown of a tooth that is impacted and enable its correct positioning on the arch through orthodontic movement.

Loss of Interdental Papilla

No technique can predictably restore a lost interdental papilla (Blatz et al. 1999; Kaushik et al. 2014). The best way to restore a papilla is not to lose it in the first place.

FACTORS THAT AFFECT THE OUTCOME OF PERIODONTAL PLASTIC PROCEDURES

Teeth Irregularity

Abnormal tooth alignment is a major cause of gingival deformities that require corrective surgery and is a significant factor in determining the outcomes of treatment. The location of the gingival margin, the width of the attached gingiva, and the alveolar bone height and thickness are all affected by tooth alignment.

On teeth that are tilted or rotated labially, the labial bony plate is thinner and located farther apically than on the adjacent teeth. The gingiva is receded, subsequently exposing the root. On the lingual surface of such teeth, the gingiva is bulbous and the bone margins are closer to the cemento-enamel junction (Bowers 1963; Andlin-Soboki & Bodin 1993). The level of gingival attachment on root surfaces and the width of the attached gingiva following mucogingival surgery are affected as much, or more, by tooth alignments as by variations in treatment procedures.

Orthodontic correction is indicated when performing mucogingival surgery on malpositioned teeth in an attempt to widen the attached gingiva or to restore the gingiva over denuded roots. If orthodontic treatment is not feasible, the prominent tooth should be ground to within the borders of the alveolar bone, avoiding pulp injury.

Roots covered with thin bony plates present a hazard in mucogingival surgery. Even the simplest type of flap (partial thickness) creates the risk of bone resorption on the periosteal surface (Hangorsky & Bissada 1980). Resorption in amounts that generally are not significant may cause loss of bone height when the bony plate is thin or tapered at the crest.

Mental Nerve

The mental nerve emerges from the mental foramen, most commonly apical to the first and second mandibular premolars, and usually divides into three branches. One branch turns forward and downward to the skin of the chin. The other two branches travel forward and upward to supply the skin and mucous membrane of the lower lip and the mucosa of the labial alveolar surface.

Trauma to the mental nerve can produce uncomfortable paresthesia of the lower lip, from which recovery is slow. Familiarity with the location and appearance of the mental nerve reduces the likelihood of injuring it.

Muscle Attachments

Tension from high muscle attachments interferes with mucogingival surgery by causing postoperative reduction in vestibular depth and width of the attached gingiva.

Mucogingival Junction

Ordinarily, the mucogingival line in the incisor and canine area is located approximately 3 mm apically to the crest of the alveolar bone on the radicular surfaces and 5 mm interdentally (Strahan 1963). In periodontal disease and on malpositioned, disease-free teeth, the bone margin is located farther apically and may extend beyond the mucogingival line.

The distance between the mucogingival line and the cemento-enamel junction before and after periodontal surgery is not necessarily constant. After inflammation is eliminated, there is a tendency for the tissue to contract and draw the mucogingival line in the direction of the crown (Donnenfeld & Glickman 1966).

REFERENCES

Allen, E.P., Gainza, C.S., Farthing, G.G., & Newbold, D.A. (1985) Improved technique for localized ridge augmentation: A report of 21 cases. *Journal of Periodontology* 56, 195–199.

American Academy of Periodontology (1996) Consensus report: Mucogingival therapy. *Annals of Periodontology* 1, 702–706.

American Academy of Periodontology (2015) Periodontal soft tissue non-root coverage procedures: a consensus report from the AAP Regeneration Workshop. Scheyer, E.T., Sanz, M., Dibart, S., Greenwell, H., John, V., Kim, D.M., Langer, L., Neiva, R., & Rasperini, G. *Journal of Periodontology* 86(2 Suppl), 73–76.

Andlin-Sobocki, A., & Bodin, L. (1993) Dimensional alterations of the gingiva related to changes of facial/lingual tooth position in permanent anterior teeth of children. A 2-year longitudinal study. *Journal of Clinical Periodontology* 20, 219–224.

Blatz, M.B., Hurzeler, M.B., & Strub, J.R. (1999) Reconstruction of the lost interproximal papilla: presentation of surgical and nonsurgical approaches. *Periodontics and Restorative Dentistry* 19(4), 395–406.

Bowers, G.M. (1963) A study of the width of the attached gingiva. *Journal of Periodontology* 34, 201–209.

Bragger, U., Lauchenauer, D., & Lang N.P. (1992) Surgical lengthening of the clinical crown. *Journal of Clinical Periodontology* 19, 58–63.

Donnenfeld, O.W., & Glickman, I. (1966) A biometric study of the effects of gingivectomy. *Journal of Periodontology* 36, 447–452.

Edwards, J.G. (1977) The diatema, the frenum, the frenectomy: A clinical study. *American Journal of Orthodontics* 71, 489–508.

Garber, D.A., & Salama, M.A. (1996) The aesthetic smile: Diagnosis and treatment. *Periodontology 2000* 11, 18–79.

Hangorsky, U., & Bissada, N.F. (1980) Clinical assessment of free gingival graft effectiveness on the maintenance of periodontal health. *Journal of Periodontology* 51, 274–278.

Hawkins, C.H., Sterrett, J.D., Murphy, H.J., & Thomas, R.C. (1991) Ridge contour related to esthetics and function. *Journal of Prosthetic Dentistry* 66, 165–168.

Jemt, T., Book, K., Lie, A., & Borjesson, T. (1994) Mucosal topography around implants in edentulous upper jaws: Photogrammetric three-dimensional measurements of the effect of replacement of a removable prosthesis with a fixed prosthesis. *Clinical Oral Implants Research* 5, 220–228.

Kaushik, A., Pk, P., Jhamb, K., Chopra, D., Chaurasia, V.R., Masamatti, V.S., Dk, S., & Babaji, P. (2014) Clinical evaluation of papilla reconstruction using subepithelial connective tissue grafts. *Journal of Clinical and Diagnostic Research* 8(9), 77–81.

Lin, G.H., Chan, H.L., & Wang, H.L. (2013) The significance of keratinized mucosa on implant health: a systematic review. *Journal of Periodontology* 84(12), 1755–1767.

Miller, P.D. (1985) A classification of marginal tissue recession. *International Journal of Periodontics and Restorative Dentistry* 5(2), 8–13.

Murtomma, H., Meurman, J.H., Rytomaa, I., & Tutola, L. (1987) Periodontal status in university students. *Journal of Clinical Periodontology* 14(8), 462–465.

Nevins, M. (1986) Attached gingival-mucogingival therapy and restorative dentistry. *International Journal of Periodontics and Restorative Dentistry* 6(4), 9–27.

Schrott, A.R., Jimenez, M., Hwang, J.W., Fiorellini, J., & Weber, H.P. (2009) Five-year evaluation of the influence of keratinized mucosa on peri-implant soft-tissue health and stability around implants supporting full-arch mandibular fixed prostheses. *Clinical Oral Implants Research* 20(10), 1170–1177.

Seibert, J.S. (1993) Reconstruction of the partially edentulous ridge: Gateway to improved prosthetics and superior aesthetics. *Practical Periodontics and Aesthetic Dentistry* 5, 47–55.

Sharma, A., Rahul, G.R., Poduval, S.T., & Shetty, K. (2012) Short clinical crowns: treatment considerations and techniques. *Journal of Clinical Experimental Dentistry* 14(4), 230–236.

Sonick, M. (1997) Esthetic crown lengthening for maxillary anterior teeth. *Compendium of Continuing Education in Dentistry* 18(8), 807–812.

Strahan, J.D. (1963) The relation of the mucogingival junction to the alveolar bone margin. *Dental Practitioner and Dental Record* 14, 72–74.

Wennstrom, J.L. (1996) Mucogingival therapy. *Annals of Periodontology* 1, 671–701.

Yeh, S., & Andreana, S. (2004) Crown lengthening: basic principles, indications, techniques and clinical case reports. *New York State Dental Journal* 70(8), 30–36.

Chapter 2 Surgical Armamentarium, Sutures, Anesthesia, and Postoperative Management

Serge Dibart

ARMAMENTARIUM

This includes the basic surgical kit:

- Mouth mirror
- Periodontal probe (UNC 15; Hu-Friedy, Chicago, IL, USA)
- College pliers (DP2; Hu-Friedy)
- Scalpel handle no. 5 (Hu-Friedy) with blade no. 15 or 15C
- Tissue pliers (TPKN; Hu-Friedy)
- Periosteal elevator 24G (Hu-Friedy)
- Prichard periosteal elevator (PR-3; Hu-Friedy)
- Gracey curette 11/12 or Younger-Good universal curette (Hu-Friedy)
- Rhodes back-action periodontal chisel (Hu-Friedy)
- Castroviejo needle holder (Hu-Friedy)
- Goldman-Fox curved scissors (Hu-Friedy)
- A 5-0 silk suture with P-3 needle
- A 5-0 chromic gut suture with C-3 needle
- Periodontal dressing

For basic microsurgical procedures, add the following to the kit:

- Magnifying loupes ×4 (or higher) wide field or surgical microscope
- Surgical headlight (optional)
- Miniblade scalpel handle with miniblades (round tip and spoon blade angle of 2.5 mm)
- Micro Castroviejo needle holder
- Castroviejo curved microsurgical scissors
- Microsurgical tissue pliers

- A 6-0 chromic gut suture with C-1 needle
- A 7-0 coated vicryl suture 3/8 with 6.6-mm needle

SUTURES

Use the smallest and least reactive suture material compatible with the surgical problem (Halstead 1913).

Types

Two major categories of suture materials exist—resorbable and nonresorbable. These sutures are best used with tapercut needles, which have a sharp point and pass atraumatically through the mucogingival tissue, making them ideal for periodontal plastic surgery use.

Nonresorbable Sutures

Silk (Braided)

A silk suture is easy to use, and its smooth handling ensures knot security. A disadvantage, however, is that it will absorb plaque and may infect the wound if kept longer than 1 week.

Polyester (Nylon Monofilament, Polytetrafluoroethylene)

The polyester suture can be kept in the mouth longer, for 2–3 weeks, with little risk of infection. A disadvantage is that it is likely to untie if extreme care is not exerted when tying the knot. This is a result of the materials' characteristics.

Resorbable Sutures

Gut

A gut suture has mild tensile strength and is resorbed by the body's enzymes in approximately 5–7 days. A disadvantage is that its knot-handling properties are inferior to those of silk sutures. Gut sutures may untie, so care must be taken not to cut the ends too short. Gut sutures may also irritate the tissues.

Practical Periodontal Plastic Surgery, Second Edition. Edited by Serge Dibart.
© 2017 John Wiley & Sons, Inc. Published 2017 by John Wiley & Sons, Inc.

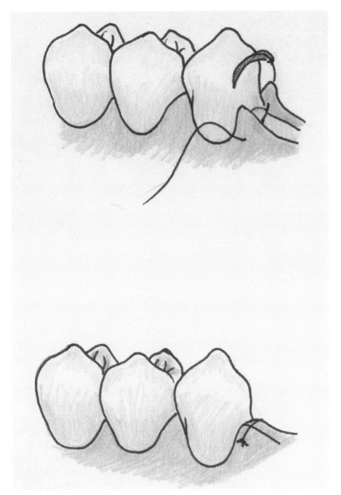

Figure 2.1 Single interrupted suture.

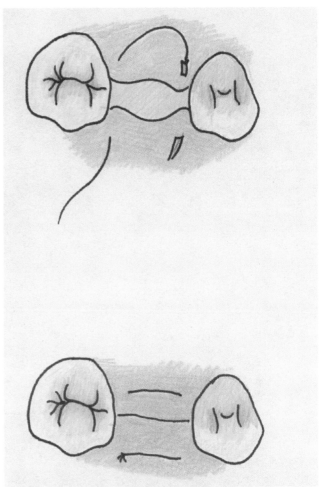

Figure 2.2 Horizontal mattress sutures.

Chromic Gut

A chromic gut suture has moderate tensile strength and is resorbed in 7–10 days. This suture is more practical than the gut suture.

Polyglycolic Acid (Synthetic)

The polyglycolic acid suture has good tensile strength, resorbs slowly (within 3–4 weeks intraorally), and is broken down through slow hydrolysis.

Sizes

Suture sizes vary from 1-0 to 10-0, with 10-0 being the thinnest. The most common size used for periodontal plastic macrosurgery is 5-0, and the most common sizes used for periodontal microsurgery are 6-0, 7-0, and 8-0.

Cyanoacrylates (Butyl and Isobutyl Forms)

Cyanoacrylate sutures have been used in wound closure since the mid-1960s. The cyanoacrylates can cement tissues together and dissolve in 4–7 days (McGraw & Caffesse 1978).

These sutures should not be used alone to secure wound closure, but can be used as an adjunct to sutures.

Techniques

- Single interrupted suture (Fig. 2.1)
- Horizontal mattress suture (Fig. 2.2)
- Vertical mattress suture (Fig. 2.3)
- Crisscross suture (Fig. 2.4)
- Sling suture (Fig. 2.5)

ANESTHESIA

Most of the time, adequate and profound anesthesia for soft tissue resection and limited bone contouring may be secured through infiltration. Block anesthesia may reduce the number of needle punctures in nonanesthetized tissue, but infiltration will achieve tissue rigidity and hemostasis that are useful when proceeding with the incisions.

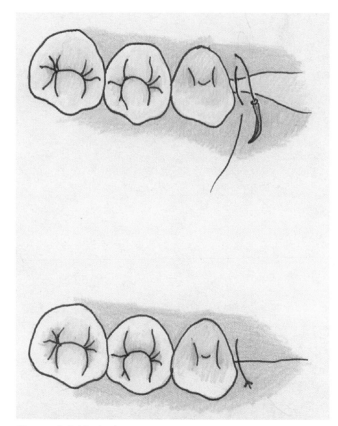

Figure 2.3 Vertical mattress suture.

Necessary Armamentarium

- 10 ml chlorhexidine gluconate 0.12
- Topical anesthetic and application tip
- Anesthetic aspirating syringe
- 30-gauge needle
- Lidocaine hydrochloride (HCl) with 1/100,000 epinephrine
- Lidocaine HCl with 1/50,000 epinephrine (to control hemorrhaging only)

Technique

After the patient rinses for 1 min with 10 ml of chlorhexidine gluconate, dry the areas to be anesthetized with a gauze. Using a Q-tip, apply the topical anesthetic on the oral tissues for 3 min for superficial anesthesia. Then anesthetize locally using one or two carpules of lidocaine HCl with 1/100,000 epinephrine in infiltration. Distraction techniques, such as gently pressing the tissues at some distance of the intended puncture site, may help further diminish the perception of puncture pain.

The first step is to administer the injection to the vestibular fold and then inject small amounts of anesthetic into the interdental papillae of the surgical site (buccal and palatal/lingual). You

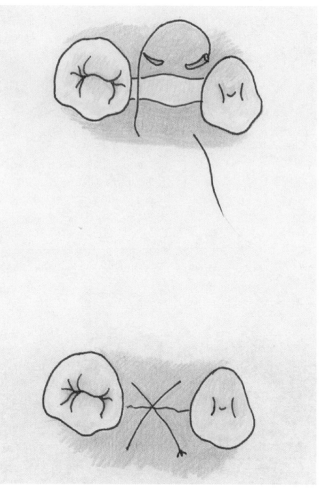

Figure 2.4 Crisscross suture.

will observe blanching of the papilla being anesthetized, the marginal gingiva, and the adjacent papilla. This will help provide a painless anesthesia as you move along the area to be anesthetized.

Diffuse the anesthetic by gently massaging the soft tissues of the vestibular fold with your finger. This will reduce the swelling occasioned by the anesthetic solution. At this time, you will be able to see your anatomical landmarks again. Massaging the tissue will also promote their rapid anesthesia.

A few drops of lidocaine HCl with 1/50,000 epinephrine can be used to control bleeding by infiltrating the tissues around the surgical site.

POSTOPERATIVE INSTRUCTIONS, MEDICATIONS, AND REGIMEN

After the procedure, the patient is given a mild analgesic while still in the office (i.e., ibuprofen 600 mg) as well as an ice pack.

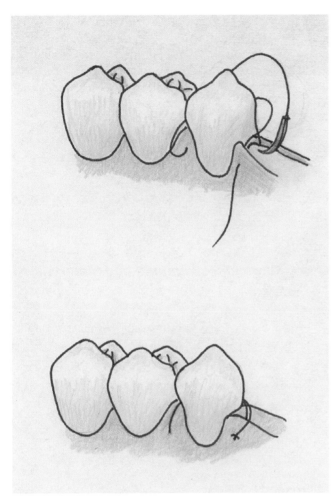

Figure 2.5 Sling suture.

Prescription

1. Ibuprofen 600 mg (Motrin) or acetaminophen 300 mg and codeine phosphate 30 mg (Tylenol no. 3) 3–4 times a day as needed for pain.

2. Chlorhexidine gluconate 0.12% to be used after week 1. Rinse twice a day for 7 days.

Instructions

Instruct the patient to keep the ice on the face for the next 2 h, 20 min on and 20 min off. Also instruct the patient to keep a soft diet and to avoid alcoholic beverages and hot or spicy food for the next 48 h. The patient should also refrain from rinsing, physical exercise, and taking drugs containing aspirin.

The sutures, if nonresorbable, will be removed after 1 week, and the patient will be asked to rinse with chlorhexidine gluconate 1.2% for 1 week after the removal of the sutures.

Specific Instructions After Soft Tissue Grafting

Emphasize to the patient that the 4 days following the surgery are critical for the success of the graft. It should be remembered that, when transplanted, a diffusion system will maintain both the graft's epithelium and connective tissue for approximately 3 days until circulation is restored (Foman 1960); therefore, complete immobility of the graft is a must for a successful outcome of the procedure. After suture removal, the patient should not brush the grafted area for 2 weeks. Two weeks after surgery a Q-tip, dipped in chlorhexidine gluconate, should be used in lieu of a toothbrush to clean the teeth of the grafted site. The patient should continue this for 2 months. After a 2-month period, gentle brushing of the area can be initiated.

REFERENCES

Foman, S. (1960) *Cosmetic Surgery*. Philadelphia: Lippincott, 161–200.

Halstead, W.S. (1913) Ligature and suture material. *Journal of the American Medical Association* 60, 119–125.

McGraw, V., & Caffesse, R. (1978) Cyanoacrylates in periodontics. *Journal of the Western Society of Periodontology/Periodontal Abstracts* 26, 4–13.

Chapter 3 Introduction to Microsurgery and Training

Ming Fang Su and Yu-Chuan Pan

INTRODUCTION

In 1960, J.H. Jacobson and E.L. Suarez first introduced microsurgical technique when they anastomosed small vessels under an operative microscope. In 1963, Chen Zong-Wei, the authoritative figure in microsurgery in China, reported the world's first successful replantation of an amputated forearm (Chen et al. 1963a & b). Thereafter, with the development and refinement of microsurgical technique and its clinical application, much progress has been made in reconstructive surgery throughout the world.

TRAINING IN MICROSURGERY

Generally speaking, microsurgery techniques are comparatively difficult to learn. Learning microsurgical skills requires practice that involves a period of hardship and endurance. Before the clinical application in patients, it is paramount that one trains in the laboratory and on animal models to gain familiarity with techniques.

Since viewing objects under the microscope or surgical loupes is different from viewing objects with the naked eye, a surgeon's hand–eye coordination must be precisely adjusted according to various degrees of magnification. The hands must be trained for delicate manipulation. This is one of the challenges in microsurgery. The higher the magnification is, the more accurate the maneuvering that is required.

BASIC MICROINSTRUMENTATION

Few items are required for training in microsurgery (Fig. 3.1).

Microsurgery Basic Set

The five pieces are:

- One curved, 14-m-long microneedle holder
- Two straight, 15-cm-long micro-strong forceps, with a 0.3-mm tip and round handle with platform

- One straight, 14-cm-long forceps, with a 0.2-mm tip and round handle with platform
- One straight, 14-cm-long scissors

Other Surgical Instruments and Materials

These include:

- Straight, 12.5-cm-long Adson forceps (Microsurgery Instruments, Bellaire, TX, USA), with 1 × 2 teeth
- Curved, 12.5-cm-long Iris scissors (Microsurgery Instruments)
- Suture card with 16 lines for suture practice
- Vascular double clamps
- Irrigating needle and spring

Microneedle Holder

The needle holder is used to grasp the needle, pull it through the tissues, and tie knots. The needle should be held between its middle and lower thirds at its distal tip. If the needle is held too close to the top, the anastomosis between the two ends of the vessel cannot be completed with a single stitch. If it is held too close to the bottom, maintaining steady control is difficult, and the direction of the tip can be changed easily. The needle can be bent or broken if too much force is used.

The needle holder is mainly manipulated by the thumb, index, and middle fingers, similar to how a pencil is held between the fingers. With this pencil-holding posture, the hand is maintained in a functional or neutral position.

The appropriate needle-holder length depends on the nature of the operation. The most commonly used are 14 cm and 18 cm. The tips can be straight or gently curved, but the latter are most often used. The choice of the tip is determined by the nature of the suture. Usually a delicate tip (0.3 mm) is used for 8-0 and 10-0 sutures. The needle holder with a 1-mm tip is used for 5-0 and 6-0 sutures.

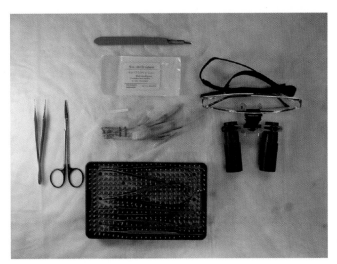

Figure 3.1 Basic setup for microsurgical training, including a chicken's foot (see text).

Dentists commonly use a locking-type needle holder. A locking needle holder is useful because one can hold the needle securely, which is most important during needle insertion. To minimize jogging, the lock should be closed slowly but released promptly. Dedicated practice is necessary to develop skillful manipulation of the needle holder.

A needle holder should ensure that a needle is held steadily without slipping. It should be light and require the minimal force from the hand. It should be a length to suit the size of the hand and be manipulated easily. A titanium needle holder is the best choice.

Microforceps

These are important instruments in microsurgery, especially for delicate manipulation and detailed movement. They are used to handle minute tissues without damaging them and to hold fine sutures while tying knots. Microforceps can make those maneuvers that cannot be performed by hand. For example, the forceps can be inserted into the lumen of a cut vessel end to open the vascular lumen for needle insertion. The forceps used for vessel anastomosis are very fine and called *dilators*.

A standard pair of forceps should be able to pick up a 100 nylon suture on a glass board without slipping. The tips of the forceps should be smooth and strong. The forceps should not damage the tissue, and no break to the suture should occur during suturing.

Microdissection

Microforceps are used for dissection, especially for blood vessels and nerves. A common mistake occurs when the tips of the forceps adhere to the vessel wall, and the vessel breaks, which

leads to massive bleeding. Therefore, when using the forceps for dissection, the artery and the vein should not be touched with the tips, which should be kept closed. The sides of the tips are used for dissection of tissues and blood vessels, similar to how fingers are used during blunt dissection in general surgery.

To prevent unnecessary bleeding, it is important to remember to use the *sides* of the tips for dissection so that the tips do not face and break the vessels. Delicate dissection can be performed after one is familiar with the use of microforceps. Even 0.3- to 0.5-mm blood vessels or nerves can be handled after repeated practice.

There are different types of microforceps for different operations. The most commonly used microforceps are 15 cm long, with round handles and 0.2- to 0.3-mm tips. The rounded handle enables the direction, degree, and position of the instrument to be changed by merely rolling the fingers, which facilitates knotting and dissection. The tips for microforceps can be straight or curved. Some have teeth to strengthen the opposing force of the tips, and some also have platforms. When operating on deeper structures, like the posterior part of the oral cavity, 18-cm-long forceps are used for dissection and for tying knots.

Jeweler forceps are strong and cheap, with a variety of tips available. They can be straight or curved at different degrees, such as 45° or 90°. They are usually 11–12 cm long and suitable only for superficial operations. Their handles are flat, which makes rotating and changing the direction of the instrument less efficient.

While stitching with a needle holder and forceps, the needle sometimes isn't in the microscopic field of view. Two different methods are adopted to find the missing needle. The first is to place the needle within the operating field under the microscope after every stitch. This is not only the easiest method but also the most time efficient. In the other method, the forceps are used to grasp one end of the thread, which slides through the tips of the forceps. The needle holder can catch the thread while the needle is seen. This should be done under the microscope to reduce operating time.

Microscissors

These are used for the dissection of tissues, blood vessels, and nerves. Different sizes of scissors are used for cutting sutures or tissue, removing adventitial tissue of vessels or nerves, and trimming vessels or nerves during repair.

The most commonly used microscissors are 14 cm and 18 cm long. To manage the delicate part of the adventitial tissues, 9-cm microscissors are preferable.

The tips of the scissor blades can be straight or gently curved. Straight scissors cut sutures and trim the adventitia of vessels or nerve endings. Curved scissors dissect vessels and nerves. The tips of the scissors should be sharp and cut with ease. During dissection of tissues and vessels, apart from using the tips to cut, the sides of the scissors can be used for dissection with the tips closed, similar to dissection with forceps. If done properly, this is a safe and fast way to use the tips of the scissors for dissection.

Surgical Loupes

Since the mid-1960s, surgical loupes have been widely applied in microsurgery. In addition to the conventional role in pedicle dissection and flap elevation, they are also used in digital replantation, free jejunal transfer, and animal experimentation (Peters et al. 1971; McManammy 1983; Jurkiewicz 1984; Lee 1985; Shenaq et al. 1995).

Because of the exponential growth of the development of surgical loupes, those with a magnification of 2.5- to 4-fold and 5.5- to 8-fold are available.

The advantages of surgical loupes are that they are small, easy to carry, efficient, and cost-effective. If operating on a blood vessel of 1-mm diameter or larger with surgical loupes, the result will be the same as when working under a microscope. The most commonly used magnifications are 3.5- to 6.5-fold. A disadvantage of loupes is the limited magnifying power.

There are generally two types of surgical loupes:

Galilean Loupes

These, which are economical and simple to use, consist of two to three lenses and are easy to operate, light, and inexpensive. Their disadvantages are limited magnification (2.5- or 3.5-fold) and a blurry peripheral border of the visual field.

Prism Loupes (or Wide-Field Loupes)

Each of the prism loupes, which are high quality and precise, consists of seven lenses. The magnification can reach from 3.5-fold to 10-fold, and the visual field is much clearer and sharper than with other loupes.

Properties of Ideal Surgical Loupes

These include:

- Light weight: No pressure is felt on the nose bridge while wearing these loupes
- Advanced optic lenses: These have a clearer image, wider field of view, sharper picture, and a greater depth of visual field

- Vertical and interpupillary adjustment: This enables the operation to be performed with a comfortable posture
- Magnification (range, 2.5- to 8-fold) and working distances (range, 14–22 inches)
- Mounting choice: Spectacle frames and headband
- Low cost

The usual magnification of loupes for a general dentist is 2.5- to 3.5-fold. However, the magnification for a periodontist is 3.5- to 4.5-fold. Operation on delicate tissues requires loupes with a magnification of 5.5- to 6.5-fold.

Practice

It is an important step in practice to choose a pair of surgical loupes of appropriate magnification and comfortable working distance.

Proper Wear

While wearing surgical loupes, along with adjusting interpupillary and vertical distances, the band of the surgical loupes must be fixed with appropriate tightness. If the band is too tight, too much force will be exerted on the nose bridge and the head, which is uncomfortable. Pain over the nose and head, and even swelling of the soft tissue, can occur after prolonged operations if the band is too tight.

Once the band length has been appropriately adjusted, the loupes should be moved up and down 1 cm over the nose. Properly fitted loupes exert no pressure on the nose.

Adjusting the interpupillary and vertical distances for head-mounted bend loupes is necessary. The closer the lenses are to the eyes, the larger is the field of view. A comfortable size of bend is also mandatory.

Focus

Focus is the primary aim for using surgical loupes properly. If the loupes are in focus, a clear operating view is obtained, facilitating the procedure. The focus is achieved by moving the head forward and backward until the head position can be maintained.

To obtain the proper focus, repeated exercises in head and neck positioning are needed. A simple way of doing this is to use a pair of surgical loupes to read newspapers or books. After practicing this 20–30 times every day for 3–5 days, it is easier to use loupes during microsurgery. To keep the loupes in focus during reading, the muscles of the head and the neck must be trained to maintain the head position. Once this is achieved, surgical loupes can be efficiently used during operations.

SUTURING TECHNIQUES

For suturing in microsurgery, microsutures from 8-0 to 11-0 are used. The largest sutures used in current microsurgical techniques, 8-0 sutures, are often chosen for use by novices; 9-0 sutures are used for 1- to 2-mm-vessel anastomosis; 10-0 sutures are used to repair small arteries or veins with a nerve diameter of less than 1 mm; and 11-0 sutures, the least commonly used, are reserved for special situations.

Suture Card

This device used to practice suturing is made of silicon rubber or plastic and divided into 16 squares. Incisions are made on the silicon sheet in each square. A total of 16 suture lines are incised at four different directions, and 20–24 stitches are required to complete each suture line.

A total of more than 350 stitches can be made in each suture card. Different sized sutures can be practiced on this card to refine technique (Fig. 3.2).

The number of stitches made on a single suture card is equivalent to 1 year of experience of a surgeon practicing microsurgery. The reasoning behind this, for example, is that in a general hospital a plastic surgeon handles two cases of microsurgery each month and two anastomoses for each case, one for artery and one for vein. Four anastomoses are then made during each month, and each anastomosis takes eight stitches. In 1 month, 32 stitches are made and in 1 year, 384 stitches are sutured. That is equivalent to the total on a single suture card.

Quality Stitching

There is much emphasis not only on the quantity of the sutures, but also the quality. A quality stitch is required for each suture. Several requirements must be fulfilled when a stitch is made.

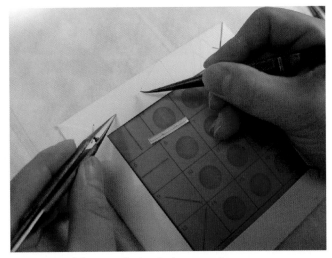

Figure 3.2 Microsurgical suturing exercise.

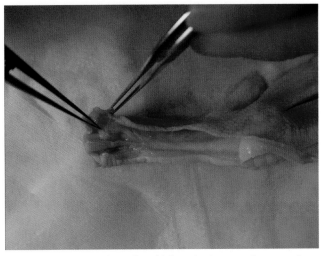

Figure 3.3 Dissection of a chicken foot, exposing an artery, a tendon, and a vein.

First, stitches should be exactly 90° to the incisions. Second, every stitch should be the same size. If the size of the stitches differs, the smoothness of the interior surface of the vessel cannot be maintained. This results in clot formation and leads to thrombosis. Third, the entry site and the exit site of every stitch should be the same width. Finally, the stitches should be equally spaced. Leaking may occur if the spacing of the stitches is uneven.

AN ANIMAL MODEL FOR MICROSURGERY TECHNIQUE TRAINING

During the training for microsurgery, every trainee has to learn the technique for tying, transplanting, and repairing different vessels, nerves, and tissue. Beginners have to practice on experimental animals to acquire the skill. The chicken leg is an effective and useful microsurgical teaching model (Fig. 3.3).

A chicken leg is a composite tissue with skin, fascia, muscle, nerve, artery, vein, and bone. It is a convenient and useful practicing material for a beginner in microsurgery, and is also readily available in supermarkets. To begin, the chicken leg is fixed on a wooden board with tape. The skin at the back is cut open to expose the fascia, muscles, nerves, and vessels. The artery length is 2–2.5 cm, with a diameter of 1.5 mm. Anastomosis can be performed up to three times on an artery. The diameter of a vein is 2–3 mm.

The openings for the artery and the vein are located at the back of the knee joint. They are both underneath the fascia and at the edge of the muscle, which can be observed with ease using surgical loupes or a microscope. The tissue is vertically dissected underneath the fascia with a pair of scissors to expose the artery, which is a pink figure beside the nerve. This blood vessel is suitable for practicing anastomosis, familiarizing oneself with the operation of a microscope or surgical loupes with 5.5- to 6.5-fold magnification, and coordinating hand–eye movements. Dye may be injected into an anastomosed vessel to assess the patency and observe any leakage. Training may continue on the chicken's fascial tissue, nerve, vein, and bone.

Once 30–50 anastomoses have been completed, one's skills and technique will have greatly improved.

REFERENCES

Chen, Z.-W., et al. (1963a) Replantation of an amputated forearm. *Chinese Journal of Surgery* 11, 767.

Chen, Z.-W., Chen, Y.C., & Pao, Y.S. (1963b) Salvage of the forearm following complete amputation: Report of a case. *Chinese Medical Journal* 82, 632.

Jacobson, J.H., & Suarez, E.L. (1960) Microsurgery in anastomosis of small vessels [Abstract]. *Surgical Forum* 11, 243–245.

Jurkiewicz, M.J. (1984) Reconstructive surgery of the cervical esophagus. *Journal of Thoracic Surgery* 88, 893–897.

Lee, S. (1985) Historical Review of Microsurgery. In: Lee, S., ed. *Manual of Microsurgery*. Boca Raton, FL: CRC, 1–3.

McManammy, D.S. (1983) Comparison of microscope and loupe magnification: Assistance for the repair of median and ulnar nerves. *British Journal of Plastic Surgery* 36, 367–372.

Peters, C.R., McKee, D.M., & Berry, B.E. (1971) Pharyngoesophageal reconstruction with revascularized jejunal transplants. *American Journal of Surgery* 121, 675–678.

Shenaq, S.M., Klebuc, M.J.A., & Vargo, D. (1995) Free-tissue transfer with the aid of loupe magnification: Experience with 251 procedures. *Plastic and Reconstructive Surgery* 95, 261–269.

Chapter 4 Periodontal Microsurgery

James Belcher

HISTORICAL PERSPECTIVE

References to magnification date back 2800 years, when simple glass meniscus lenses were described in ancient Egyptian writings. In 1694, Amsterdam merchant Anton van Leeuwenhook constructed the first compound-lens microscope. Magnification for microsurgical procedures was introduced to medicine during the late 1800s. In 1921, Carl Nylen, who is considered the father of microsurgery, first used the binocular microscope for ear surgery (Dohlman 1969). It was not until 1960, when Jacobsen and Suarez obtained 100% patency in suturing 1-mm-diameter blood vessels for anastomosis, that the surgical microscope gained wide acceptance in medicine (Barraquer 1980).

Apotheker & Jako (1981) first introduced the microscope to dentistry in 1978. During 1992, Carr published an article outlining the use of the surgical microscope during endodontic procedures. In 1993, Shanelec & Tibbetts (1998) presented a continuing education course on periodontal microsurgery at the annual meeting of the American Academy of Periodontology. This led to centers devoted to teaching periodontists and other dentists periodontal microsurgery.

Belcher wrote an article in 2001 summarizing the benefits and potential usages of the surgical microscope in periodontal therapy. Although Belcher and several other periodontists view the addition of the microscope as invaluable in periodontal therapy, it has been cautiously accepted by the periodontal profession as a whole.

PERIODONTAL APPLICATIONS

The operating microscope offers three distinct advantages to periodontists: illumination, magnification, and increased precision of surgical skills (Belcher 2001). The synergy of improved illumination and increased visual acuity enables the increased precision of surgical skills. Collectively, these advantages can be referred to as the *microsurgical triad* (Fig. 4.1).

Among many basic surgical principles, several are germane to periodontal surgery. Eliminating dead space, tissue handling, removal of necrotic tissue and foreign materials, closure with sufficient but appropriate tension, and immobilization of the wound are important surgical goals in periodontal therapy (Johnson & Johnson 1994, p. 9). The surgical operating microscope and appropriate microsurgical technique afford surgeons a more realistic chance of achieving these goals.

In periodontics, the surgical operating microscope, though useful in most areas of periodontal therapy, is particularly useful in mucogingival surgery, root preparation, and crown-lengthening procedures.

Microsurgical techniques are especially beneficial to mucogingival procedures on natural teeth and implants. As mentioned above, the principles of wound healing require minimal dead space. The microscope enables clinicians to use smaller needles, sutures, and instruments, and precisely position tissues and stabilize the mending tissues.

Root preparation is an important modality in periodontal therapy. Lindhe & Nyman (1984) have suggested that the success of periodontal therapy is due to the thoroughness of debridement of the root surface. Data show that surgical access improves the ability to remove calculus (Cobb 1996). Furthermore, research demonstrates that root preparation is enhanced when performed under illumination (Reinhardt et al. 1985). The surgical microscope provides fiber optic lighting and magnification for calculus removal.

Most published articles embracing the benefits of magnification in dentistry have been anecdotal (Campbell 1989). However, two articles do show enhanced clinical benefits of magnification. Leknius & Geissberger (1995) have shown a direct relationship between magnification and significantly enhanced performance of prosthodontic dental procedures.

A recently published article concluded that performing root-coverage techniques microsurgically versus macrosurgically substantially improved the vascularization of connective tissue grafts and the percentage of additional root coverage (Burdhardt & Lang 2005). There is a lack of studies in dentistry comparing the benefits of crown lengthening or other surgical procedures via standard versus microsurgical methods. Yet it seems logical that if magnification is beneficial in prosthetics

Practical Periodontal Plastic Surgery, Second Edition. Edited by Serge Dibart.
© 2017 John Wiley & Sons, Inc. Published 2017 by John Wiley & Sons, Inc.

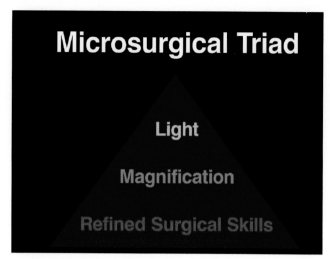

Figure 4.1 Microsurgical triad.

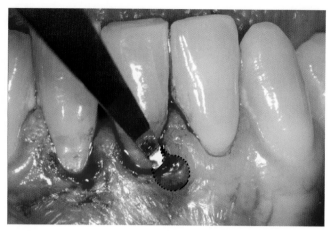

Figure 4.3 Spoon knife shown in sulcular undermining incision.

and root coverage, the surgical microscope, with its magnification, would aid practitioners in crown lengthening, root preparation, and other periodontal surgical procedures.

PERIODONTAL INSTRUMENTATION

Magnification enables dentists to use smaller instrumentation with more precision. Although the variety of microsurgical instrumentation designed for periodontal therapy is vast, the instrumentation can be divided into the following subgroups: knives, retractors, scissors, needle holders, tying forceps, and others.

The knives most commonly used in periodontal microsurgery are those used in ophthalmic surgery: blade breaker, crescent, minicrescent, spoon, lamella, and scleral knives (Fig. 4.2). The common characteristics of these knives are their extreme sharpness and small size. This enables precise incisions and maneuvers in small areas (Fig. 4.3).

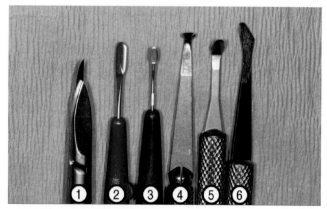

Figure 4.2 Periodontal microsurgical knives: 1, blade breaker; 2, crescent; 3, minicrescent; 4, 260° spoon; 5, lamella, and 6, sclera.

The blade-breaker knife has a handle onto which a piece of an ophthalmic razor blade is affixed. This allows for infinite angulations of the blade. This knife is often used in place of a no. 15 blade.

The crescent knife can be used for intrasulcular procedures. It is available with one-piece handles or as a removable blade. It can be used in connective tissue graft procedures to obtain the donor graft, to tunnel under tissue, and to prepare the recipient site.

The spoon knife is beveled on one side, allowing the knife to track through the tissue adjacent to bone. It is frequently used in microsurgical procedures to undermine tissue, enhancing the placement of a connective tissue graft.

Retractors and elevators have been downsized. Scissors such as micro-vannas tissue scissors are used for removal of small fragments of tissue. Needle holders are also downsized from sizes designed for conventional periodontal surgery. Tying forceps are an essential component of two-hand microsurgical tying. They are available in two general styles: platform and nonplatform. Several designs of both needle holders and tying forceps are available.

Microsurgical instrumentation can be made with titanium or surgical stainless steel. Titanium instruments tend to be lighter, but are more prone to deformation and are usually more expensive. Stainless-steel instruments are prone to magnetization, but there is a greater number and wider variety of them.

Needles and Sutures

As mentioned earlier, basic surgical techniques are used to eliminate dead space, close a wound with sufficient but appropriate tension, and immobilize a wound (Johnson & Johnson 1994, p. 9). The appropriate combination of a properly selected

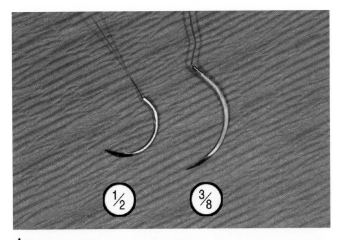

A

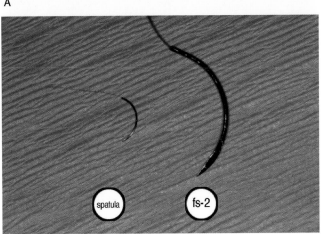

B

Figure 4.4 (A) Half-inch and three-eighths-inch curved needles. (B) Spatula needle (6.6 mm) compared to FS-2 needle (19 mm).

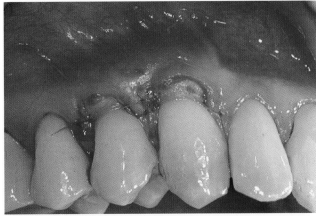

A

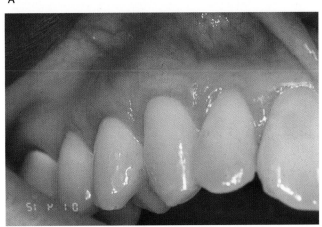

B

Figure 4.5 (A) Connective tissue graft (CTG) placement via tunnel technique. (B) Final healing of CTG.

needle and suture greatly contributes to the success of these techniques.

The most common curvature of needles used in dentistry is three-eighths of an inch (10 mm) and one-half of an inch (12.7 mm), the former being the most common (Fig. 4.4a). Dentists frequently use larger needles, such as 16–19 mm. Although larger needles are appropriate in certain surgical procedures, such as flap closure after extractions, smaller needles enable precise closure of the mending tissues in more detailed procedures.

A spatula needle, which is beneficial in periodontal microsurgical procedures, is 6.6 mm long and has a curvature of 140° (Fig. 4.4b). The combination of a shallow needle tract and precise needle purchase of the tissue enables extremely accurate apposition and closure in periodontal mucogingival surgery.

An accepted surgical practice is to use the smallest suture possible to hold the mending tissue adequately (Johnson &

Johnson 1994, p. 15). This practice minimizes the opening made by the needle and the trauma through the tissues. Frequently in periodontal microsurgical procedures, 6-0, 7-0, and 8-0 sutures are indicated.

Sutures can be classified as nonresorbable or resorbable, and can be multifilament or monofilament in design. Examples of nonresorbable sutures are silk, nylon, and polyester. Common resorbable sutures are plain and chromic gut, polyglactin 910, poliglecaprone 25, and polydioxanone. Medical studies have shown the superiority of poligle-caprone 25 and polyglactin 910 to gut (LaBabnara 1995; Anatol et al. 1997).

The combination of using smaller needles, sutures, and magnification results in minimal dead space, closure with sufficient but appropriate tension, and immobilization of the wound (Fig. 4.5).

Microsurgical Tying

Several principles of microsurgical tying are applicable to periodontal therapy: instrument grip, needle gripping, two-handed tying techniques, needle penetration, and suture guiding.

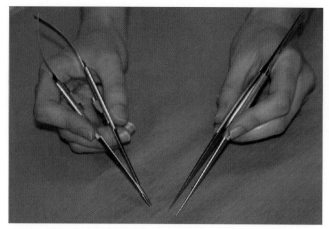

Figure 4.6 Pen grip used for microsurgical instruments.

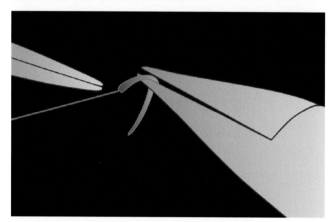

Figure 4.7 Proper gripping of needle by needle holder.

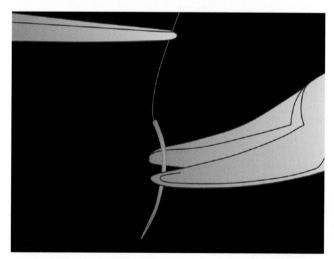

Figure 4.8 Rearming of needle.

Microsurgical instruments are most stable when held like a writing instrument (Fig. 4.6). Needles are best gripped about two-thirds down from the end of the needle (Fig. 4.7). One technique for holding the needle is to grasp the suture with tying forceps in one's nondominant hand about 2–3 cm from the needle. Dangle the needle until it rests on the tissue and grasp the needle

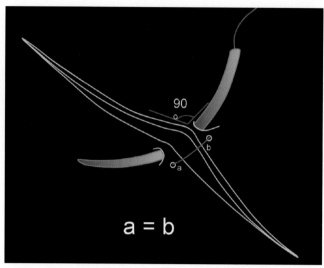

Figure 4.9 Proper entry and exit distance of needle.

with the needle holder (Fig. 4.8). The needle should be set in the needle holder pointing along the intended path.

Needle penetration should be perpendicular to the incision line. The needle should penetrate and exit the tissue at equal distances (Fig. 4.9). Depending on the needle diameter, the proper amount of tissue to engage is approximately twice that of the diameter of the needle. Engaging large amounts of tissue may not result in proper closure. The suture is best pulled through the tissue in a straight line perpendicular to the incision. Tying forceps can aid in this maneuver (Fig. 4.10).

Three common techniques are used in microsurgical tying: nondominant, dominant, and a combination of the two. These techniques are best learned in a laboratory setting and are well referenced and described in detail in *A Laboratory Manual for Microvascular and Microtubal Surgery* (Cooley 2001). The non-dominant and combination tying techniques are the two most commonly used in dentistry.

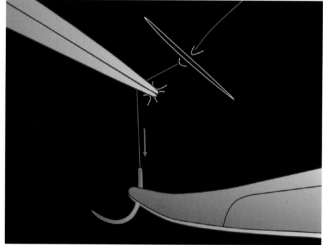

Figure 4.10 Guiding the suture direction with tying forceps.

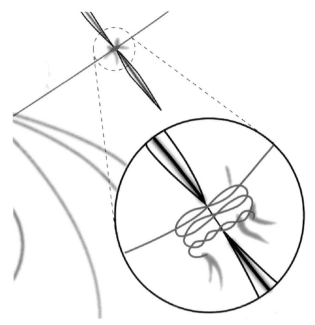

Figure 4.11 Microsurgical knot (surgeon's knot followed by square knot).

Square knots are the best to guarantee the integrity of the knot. A surgeon's knot followed by a square knot is the preferred knot combination (Fig. 4.11). Adding excess ties to a knot does not increase its strength or integrity, it only adds to the bulk of the knot.

PERIODONTAL MICROSURGICAL PROCEDURES

Mucogingival Procedures

Early attempts at root coverage included lateral flaps, free gingival grafts, and coronal advanced flaps, but the results of these methods were often unpredictable. In 1985, Raetzke published a new method for covering localized areas of root exposure described as the connective tissue graft.

A comparative summary of root-coverage studies (Greenwell et al. 2000) concluded that the connective tissue graft was the most effective and predictable method. Furthermore, another comparative study of connective tissue grafts using microsurgical and macrosurgical techniques showed substantially improved vascularization of the grafts and the percentage of root coverage compared with the conventional macroscopic approach (Burdhardt & Land 2005).

Microsurgical Techniques for Connective Tissue Grafts

Several macrosurgical techniques have been outlined in the literature for connective tissue graft recipient sites. These techniques were described as a "box" or flap (Figs. 4.12–4.14), and

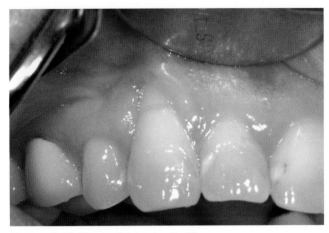

Figure 4.12 Recession on tooth #6.

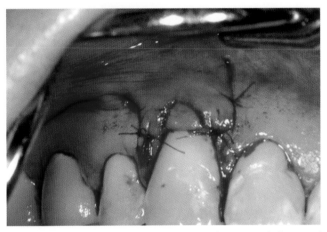

Figure 4.13 Subepithelial connective tissue graft inserted and sutured.

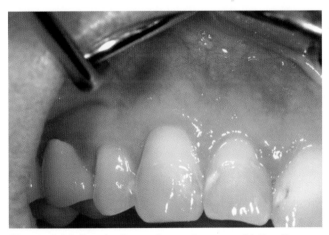

Figure 4.14 Results 3 months post surgery. Notice the perfect outcome.

sulcular and laterally positioned flaps over the connective tissue graft. Langer & Langer (1989) described one of the earlier approaches for connective tissue grafts. The refinements to this conventional procedure using microsurgical techniques allow for better positioning and closure of the incisions and, according to Burdhardt & Land (2005), better results.

Another approach to treat minimal recession is to use a sulcular, or flapless, technique. After the root is prepared with citric acid and/or tetracycline, a sulcular incision is made to detach the tissue by using a crescent knife, which, in turn, creates a pouch to receive the graft. The graft is sized at approximately 3 mm wider and longer than the recession defect and placed into the pouch.

The sling technique for microsurgical suturing is used to intimately familiarize the graft to the root surface. A 7-0 or 8-0 suture and a spatula needle are used for this portion of the procedure. The needle is first passed through the sulcus, then inverted and passed through the graft, and finally out through the interproximal tissue. As the suture is tied, the graft is tightened against the root, enabling intimate stabilization. This technique is effective in recession depths of 3 mm or less.

Numerous other microsurgical techniques can be used, such as tunnel techniques or lateral flaps covering the connective graft in more advanced recession cases (more than 3 mm). These techniques are similar to macrosurgical flap design, but are more refined because of smaller instrumentation, needles, and sutures.

MICROSURGICAL APPLICATIONS FOR IMPLANTS

Millions of dental implants are placed each year. As the numbers grow, problems such as peri-implant mucositis, perio-implantitis (Mombelli & Lang 1998), and gingival recession increasingly occur. There are numerous causes of these problems but one is an inadequately keratinized tissue around the implant neck. In a 5-year evaluation of the influence of keratinized mucosa on peri-implant soft-tissue health and stability around implants supporting full-arch mandibular fixed prostheses, the authors concluded that when keratinized mucosa is less than 2 mm, plaque accumulation increases with more soreness and more recession occurred on buccal surfaces (Shrott et al. 2009). This leads the surgeon to having to add more keratinized tissue to the implant neck and/or repair the recession.

While a clinical cohort study by Burkhardt et al. of 10 patients with peri-implant dehiscences utilizing connective tissue grafts with chronally advanced flaps and a contralateral unrestored clinical crown showed improvement at the surgical sites, complete coverage was not achieved at any treated site.

Utilizing microsurgical techniques the author has had numerous successes although the results are not as predicable as

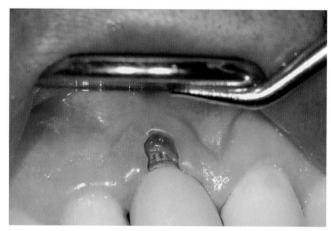

Figure 4.15 Implant replacing tooth #8 showing recession and metal collar.

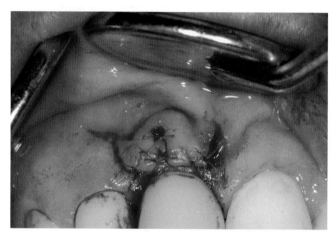

Figure 4.16 Subepithelial connective tissue graft sutured in place.

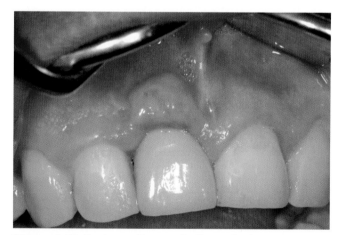

Figure 4.17 Postoperative results 2 months later.

root-coverage techniques on natural teeth (Figs. 4.15–4.17) It maybe that according to Burdhart's research the improved vascularization of the grafts can enhance the results (Burdhardt & Land 2005).

Microsurgical Applications for Root Preparation

Stereomicroscopy has often been used in dentistry to evaluate residual calculus after scaling and surgical therapy. Several researchers believe the critical determinant of successful periodontal therapy is the thoroughness of debridement of the root surface (Lindhe & Nyman 1984; Lindhe et al. 1984). Fleischer et al. (1989) stated that, regardless of the experience level of the operator, calculus-free roots were obtained more often with surgical access. Other articles comparing the amount of residual calculus on root surfaces treated by scaling and root preparation showed less residual calculus on those treated with surgical access (14–24%) than on those treated without surgical access (17–69%) (American Academy of Periodontology 1996).

Root preparation is enhanced when performed under illumination (Reinhardt et al. 1985). The surgical operating microscope is an excellent source of light. Although few studies have compared root preparation during surgical access with and without magnification, it seems logical that a surgical operating microscope would enhance a surgeon's effectiveness in root preparation.

INCORPORATING THE SURGICAL OPERATING MICROSCOPE IN PRACTICE

Microsurgical skills are not beyond the ability of dentists. We often work in small and confined places. It can require numerous hours of training to use a microscope, similar to the neurological retraining we had to accomplish to switch from direct view to indirect mirror view. Certain principles of microsurgery should to be adhered to, and one should approach training in microsurgery with a fresh and open mind. One should not approach learning the skills of microsurgery as an endurance test. Frequent breaks and recurrent training are beneficial. Certainly, controlled training at a microsurgical training facility with experienced faculty speeds up the process.

Several hurdles must be overcome in microsurgical training. Tremor or intrinsic, unwanted muscle movement is a problem all operators of the surgical microscope deal with to some degree. The consensus of experienced microsurgeons is that tremors are enhanced by sleep deprivation, physical exertion of the upper body within 24 h, recent nicotine exposure, excessive caffeine, irritation, and anxiety. One should avoid these before performing microsurgery.

Another skill that takes time to learn is depth-of-field perception. Similar to adapting to different visual clues when first wearing loupes, you will need time to adjust to the new visual field through a surgical microscope.

Unless the anterior facial teeth or gingival tissues are the targets, mirrors are extremely useful. Usually they are held further away from the teeth, and smaller sizes and bent handles will facilitate technique. One should also become skilled at the positioning of the microscope.

Documentation of procedures is possible through video and digital photography. It is beyond the scope of this chapter to inform readers of what photographic systems to use. The manufacturers of the surgical operating microscopes can aid professionals in setting up such systems.

SUMMARY

The surgical operating microscope provides practitioners with increased illumination, magnification, and an environment in which surgical skills can be refined. Clinicians have smaller instrumentation, sutures, and needles at their disposal to facilitate enhanced clinical skills. Although only a few studies show enhanced surgical outcomes, the increase in visual acuity provided by the surgical operating microscope should enhance a periodontist's delivery of surgical skills.

REFERENCES

Anatol, T.I., Roopchand, R., Holder, Y., & Shing-Hon, G. (1997) A comparison of the use of plain catgut, skin tapes and polyglactin sutures for skin closure: A prospective clinical trial. *Journal of the Royal College of Surgeons of Edinburgh* 42, 124–127.

Apotheker, H., & Jako, G.H. (1981) A microscope for use in dentistry. *Journal of Microsurgery* 3, 7–10.

Barraquer, J.I. (1980) The history of the microscope in ocular surgery. *Journal of Microsurgery* 1, 288–299.

Belcher, J.M. (2001) A perspective on periodontal microsurgery. *International Journal of Periodontology and Restorative Dentistry* 21, 191–196.

Burdhardt, R., & Land, N.P. (2005) Coverage of localized gingival recessions: Comparison of micro- and macrosurgical techniques. *Journal of Clinical Periodontology* 32, 287–293.

Burkhardt, R., Joss, A., & Lang, N. (2008) Soft tissue dehiscence coverage endossious implants – A prospective cohort study. *Clinical Oral Implants Research* 19, 451–457.

Campbell, D. (1989) Magnification is major aid to dentists … and how microdentistry's time has come! *Future of Dentistry* 4(3), 11.

Carr, G.B. (1992) Microscopes in endodontics. *Journal of California Dentistry* 20, 55–61.

Cobb, C.M. (1996) Non-surgical pocket therapy: Mechanical. *Annals of Periodontology* 1, 443–490.

Cooley, B.C. (2001) *A Laboratory Manual for Microsulcular and Microtubal Surgery*. Reading, PA: Surgical Specialties, 28–33.

Dohlman, G.F. (1969) Carl Olof Nylen and the birth of the otomicroscope and microsurgery. *Archives of Otolaryngology* 90, 813–817.

Fleischer, H.C., Mellonig, J.T., Brayer, W.K., Gray, J.L., & Barnett, J.D. (1989) Scaling and root planing efficacy in multirooted teeth. *Journal of Periodontology* 60, 402–409.

Greenwell, H., Bissada, N.F., Henderson, R.D., & Dodge, J.R. (2000) The deceptive nature of root coverage results. *Journal of Periodontology* 71, 1327–1337.

Johnson & Johnson (1994) *Wound Closure Manual*. Somerville, NJ: Ethicon.

LaBabnara, J. (1995) A review of absorbable suture materials in head and neck surgery and introduction of monocryl: A new absorbable suture. *Ear, Nose, and Throat Journal* 74, 409–416.

Langer, B., & Langer, L. (1989) Subepithelial connective tissue graft technique for root coverage. *Journal of Periodontology* 56, 715–720.

Leknius, C., & Geissberger, M. (1995) The effect of magnification on the performance of fixed prosthodontic procedures. *Journal of the California Dental Association* 23, 66–70.

Lindhe, J., & Nyman, S. (1984) Long-term maintenance of patients treated for advanced periodontal disease. *Journal of Clinical Periodontology* 11, 504–514.

Lindhe, J., Westfelt, E., Nyman, S., Socransky, S.S., & Haffajee, A.D. (1984) Long-term effect of surgical/nonsurgical treatment of periodontal disease. *Journal of Clinical Periodontology* 11, 448–458.

Mombelli, A., & Lang, N.P. (1998) The diagnosis and treatment of perio-implantitis. *Periodontal 2000* 17, 63–76.

Raetzke, P.B. (1985) Covering localized areas of root exposure employing the "envelope" technique. *Journal of Periodontology* 56, 397–402.

Reinhardt, R.A., Johnson, G.K., & Tussing, G.J. (1985) Root planing with interdental papillae reflection and fiber optic illumination. *Journal of Periodontology* 56, 721–726.

Schrott. A.R., Jimenez, M., Hwang, J.W., Fiorelini, J., & Weber, H.P. (2009) Five-year evaluation of the influence of deratinized mucosa on perio-implant soft-tissue health and stability around implants supporting full-arch mandibular fixed prostheses. *Clinical Oral Implants Research* 20(10), 1170–1177.

Tibbetts, L.S., & Shanelec, D.A. 1998. Periodontal microsurgery. *Dental Clinics of North America* 42, 339–359.

Chapter 5 Free Gingival Autograft

Serge Dibart

HISTORY

Bjorn in 1963, and Sullivan & Atkins in 1968, were the first to describe the free gingival autograft. The latter two applied the principles of plastic surgery to periodontology. The autograft was initially used to increase the amount of attached gingiva and extend the vestibular fornix. Later it was used to attempt coverage of exposed root surfaces (Sullivan & Atkins 1968; Holbrook & Ochsenbein 1983; Miller 1985). Simple and highly predictable when used to increase the amount of attached gingiva, it is also quite versatile: it can also be used over an extraction socket or osseous graft (Ellegaard et al. 1974).

INDICATIONS

Free gingival autografts are used for:

- Increasing the amount of keratinized tissue (more specifically, attached gingiva)

- Increasing the vestibular depth

- Increasing the volume of gingival tissues in edentulous spaces (preprosthetic procedures)

- Covering roots in areas of gingival recession

ARMAMENTARIUM

This includes the basic surgical kit plus the following:

- Absorbable gelatin sponge (Gelfoam; Pharmacia Upjohn, Kalamazoo, MI, USA), oxidized regenerated cellulose (Surgicel; Johnson & Johnson, New Brunswick, NJ, USA) or Avitene (Bard, Murray Hill, NJ, USA)

- Purified *n*-butyl cyanoacrylate (PeriAcryl GluStitch; Delta, BC, Canada)

- Citric acid pH 1 (40%) or 1 capsule of tetracycline hydrochloride (HCl), 250 mg, for root coverage

FREE GINGIVAL AUTOGRAFT TO INCREASE KERATINIZED TISSUE

Technique

Preparation of the Recipient Site

Using the scalpel, a no. 15 blade, trace the horizontal incision line below the gingival recession (Figs. 5.1 & 5.2). You may keep or remove the gingival sulcus. Place two vertical incisions, extending beyond the mucogingival junction, at the end of that horizontal line. Place the releasing incisions at line angles of the adjacent teeth and proceed with a partial thickness flap, leaving the periosteum on the alveolar bone.

At this stage, it is critical to dissect as close as possible to the periosteum, to remove epithelium, connective tissue, and muscle fibers, so there is as little movable soft tissue as possible. This decreases the likelihood of a movable graft after the healing process.

Once the bed has been prepared, the superficial flap can be removed using scissors. If you decide to keep the flap, it should be sutured below the graft once the graft has been secured.

Some authors advocate the placement of the graft on denuded bone (Dordick et al. 1976; James & McFall 1978), reporting less shrinkage and a firmer, less mobile graft. In this particular technique, the surgeon removes the periosteum, as well as the other structures mentioned previously, such as the epithelium, connective tissue, and muscle fibers, to expose the alveolar bone. The incisions go down to the bone, with the blade in contact with the bone, cutting the periosteum.

The full-thickness flap is then elevated with a periosteal elevator to uncover the underlying bone. This dissection is called a *blunt dissection* as opposed to the aforementioned *sharp dissection* for the partial thickness flap. If the graft is placed on denuded bone, it is important to decorticate the alveolar plate using a small round burr (no. 1/2). This enables faster revascularization of the graft via the formation of capillary outgrowths.

Practical Periodontal Plastic Surgery, Second Edition. Edited by Serge Dibart.
© 2017 John Wiley & Sons, Inc. Published 2017 by John Wiley & Sons, Inc.

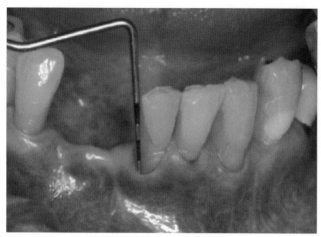

Figure 5.1 Tooth 25 had a recession and lack of attached gingiva.

Graft Harvesting From the Donor Site

It is customary to take the graft from the palate between the palatal root of the first molar and the distal line angle of the canine. This is the area where the thickest tissue can be found (Reiser et al. 1996). However, any other edentulous area, such as the edentulous ridge, attached gingiva, or accessible tuberosities, will be just as sufficient.

When harvesting the graft, it is advisable to avoid the neurovascular bundle, which includes the greater and lesser palatine nerves and blood vessels. Avoid the palatal rugae as well (Cohen 1994). The neurovascular bundle enters the palate through the greater and lesser palatine foramina, apical to the third molars, and then travels across the palate and into the incisive foramen.

Reiser et al. in 1996 reported that the neurovascular bundle could be located 7–17 mm from the cemento-enamel junction (CEJ) of the maxillary premolars and molars. According to these

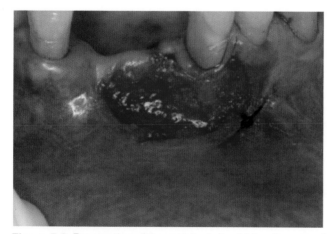

Figure 5.2 Preparation of the recipient site. A bleeding vessel has been tied with a black silk suture.

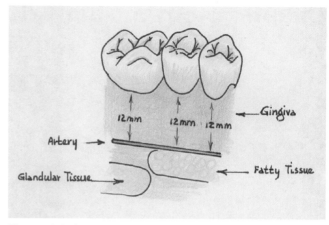

Figure 5.3 Anatomy of a donor region. Palatal vessels and nerve running from the greater and lesser palatine foramina to the interincisive foramen. The anterior palatal submucosa is mainly fatty, whereas the posterior palatal submucosa is mainly glandular.

authors, in the average palatal vault the distance from the CEJ to the neurovascular bundle is 12 mm (Fig. 5.3). That distance is shortened to 7 mm in case of a shallow palatal vault and lengthened to 17 mm in case of a high palatal vault.

Other research has shown gender-related variations. The mean height of the palatal vault, as measured from the midline of the palate to the CEJ of the first molars, is 14.90 ± 2.93 mm in men and 12.70 ± 2.45 mm in women (Redman et al. 1965).

Needle sounding while anesthetizing the area can be a useful tool in approximating the location of the palatal artery as well as the thickness of the tissues. The inclusion of palatal rugae in the graft should be avoided because it could be detrimental to aesthetics. The transplanted graft may retain its original morphology long after the procedure is done, and the rugae remain despite efforts to eliminate them surgically (Breault et al. 1999).

After measuring the denuded area with a periodontal probe at the recipient site, the measurements of the palate should be recorded and the graft outline traced with the scalpel (Fig. 5.4). The graft thickness should be close to 1.5 mm, which approximately corresponds to the length of the bevel on a no. 15 blade, and should not be too thick or too thin. The dissection is done with a no. 15 blade kept parallel to the epithelial outer side of the graft, not the long axis of the tooth.

The submucosa of the anterior palate is rich in fat (Orban 1996) and care must be taken to avoid including the fatty layer in the graft. If that layer is included, the fat is removed from the graft with the scalpel before suturing it to the recipient bed. The excision has to be atraumatic, and every effort must be made to have a smooth, even, and regular connective tissue surface (Figs. 5.5 & 5.6). This is important because it will minimize dead

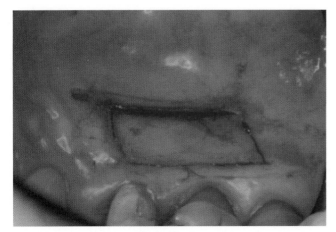

Figure 5.4 Palatal donor site. The graft to be harvested had been delineated with a no. 15 blade.

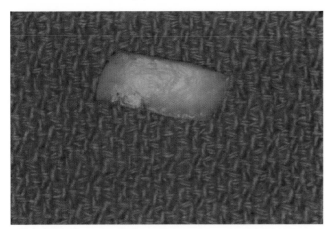

Figure 5.5 The palatal graft has been harvested.

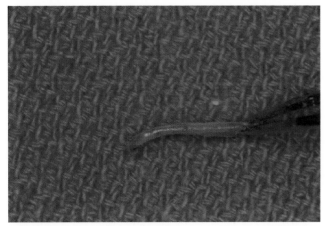

Figure 5.6 The graft is even and approximately 1.5 mm thick.

space between the graft and the recipient bed and enable quick revascularization of the graft.

Once the graft is harvested, it should be immediately sutured onto the recipient site with the connective tissue facing down against the periosteum of the recipient site.

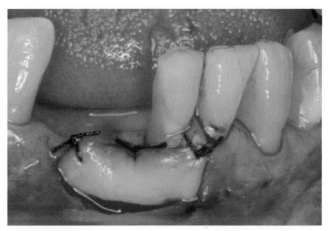

Figure 5.7 The graft is sutured in place with three single interrupted silk sutures (5-0). At this stage, when pulling on the lip, the graft should be immobile.

Graft Suturing

The use of resorbable or nonresorbable material is a matter of personal preference. Silk is easy to use but should be removed after 1 week. Gut/chromic gut, on the other hand, will resorb in 1–2 weeks. Single interrupted sutures are usually placed to secure the graft mesially and distally (Fig. 5.7). A mesiodistal horizontal suture could be added to wrap the lower half of the graft (Fig. 5.8). Variations include intraperiosteal X sutures (Fig. 5.9). They are all aimed at immobilizing the graft and decreasing the amount of dead space between recipient site and graft. This helps minimize the size of the blood clot and creates a better adaptation that will ensure prompt and proper revascularization.

Applying some pressure with wet gauze over the sutured graft for a few minutes will displace the blood under the graft, reducing hematomas, and closely position the graft to the recipient bed. Plasma will be converted to fibrin, and this fibrin clot will anchor the graft to its bed and enable rapid penetration

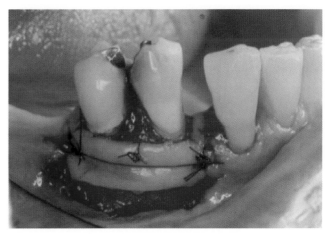

Figure 5.8 The mesiodistal horizontal suture.

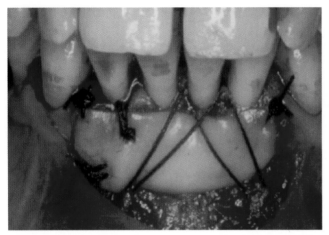

Figure 5.9 The graft is kept in place by adding two circular intraperiosteal sutures to the four single interrupted sutures present.

by capillaries. It will act as a matrix through which metabolites and waste products diffuse (Foman 1960). A good test for checking the immobility of the graft is to pull the lip or cheek gently once the graft has been sutured. If the graft moves, then the suturing or the size of the recipient bed was inadequate.

A small periodontal dressing is applied on the graft to protect the recipient site. Care must be taken when applying the dressing so it will not impinge on occlusal surfaces; otherwise, it will be lost within hours.

Donor Site

This is usually left without a dressing, so that it may granulate (Figs. 5.10 & 5.11). If the graft is large and the thickness important, it can be useful, for the comfort of the patient, to apply a piece of Gelfoam or Surgicel to the donor site and suture over it with X sutures. This is followed by an application of a few

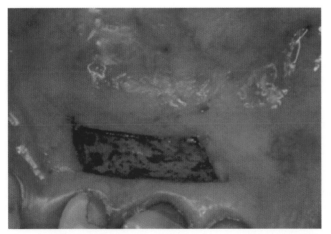

Figure 5.10 The donor site at time of surgery. The connective tissue is left exposed to granulate.

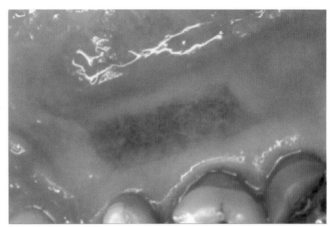

Figure 5.11 The donor site 1 week later.

drops of medical-grade cyanoacrylate glue (PeriAcryl), which will ensure hemostasis and decrease postoperative discomfort for the patient.

Graft Healing

Prior to reestablishment of vascularization (24–48 h), the graft is solely dependent on diffusion from its host bed. This diffusion, which is called *plasmic circulation*, occurs most efficiently through the fibrin clot (Foman 1960; Reese & Stark 1961). The next step is the re-establishment of graft vascularization. Capillary proliferations begin at the end of day 1, and by day 2 or 3 some capillaries have extended into the graft and others have anastomosed or penetrated the graft's vasculature. Adequate blood supply does not appear to be present until about day 8 (Davis & Traut 1925).

Concomitant with vascularization, organic connective tissue union between the graft and its bed starts on day 4 and is complete by day 10. This will be responsible for the secondary contraction of the graft. Upon healing, the graft may shrink by as much as 33% (Egli et al. 1975) (Fig. 5.12).

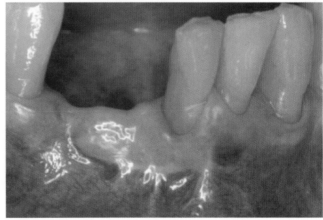

Figure 5.12 Results 2 years later. A band of attached gingival is present below and around tooth 25.

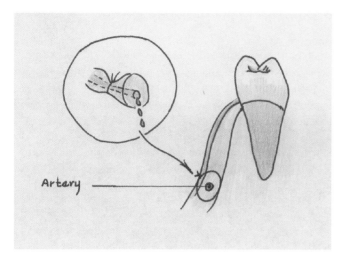
Figure 5.13 Compressive suture of the palatal artery.

Possible Complications

The main complication of the procedure is bleeding from the donor site. This can happen during the procedure or after the patient's departure from the office.

During the Procedure

Do not panic if bleeding occurs during the procedure. Assess the bleeding source (arterial versus venous) and location. If the palatal artery or a branch has been severed, it is best to place one or more compressive sutures in the palate, proximal to the bleeding site, to reduce or stop the hemorrhage (Fig. 5.13). The sutures should be placed between the bleeding site and the palatal foramina.

It is useful at this stage to use a few drops of Xylocaine (lidocaine) 2% with 1/50,000 epinephrine in infiltration around the bleeding area to help with the hemostasis. Finish the grafting procedure, cover the donor site with Gelfoam or Surgicel, and secure with an X suture. Use compression with wet gauze for 5–10 min and finish by applying a few drops of PeriAcryl over the donor site.

Another alternative is to cauterize the bleeding vessel. As a last resort, some authors have advocated the elevation of a full-thickness flap to enable the visualization and ligation of the blood vessels (Hollingshead 1968).

After the Procedure

If bleeding occurs after the procedure, assure the patient of his or her safety. Have the patient moisten a tea bag and ask him or her to put the tea bag on the palate and press on it for 10–15 min. If the bleeding does not stop, ask the patient to come to your office. Once in the office, use the aforementioned procedure—infiltration with lidocaine 2% with 1/50,000 epinephrine, compressive sutures, Gelfoam, etc.—or send the patient to an emergency room.

Other Complications

Swelling and Bruising

Another complication of the procedure may include swelling and bruising at the recipient site. After the initial use of cold pad within the first 24 h, the application of warm pads, in conjunction with anti-inflammatory medications, will ease the problem.

Graft Mobility

Graft mobility after complete healing is usually the result of improper bed preparation. Too much loose tissue or muscle fibers left above the periosteum will result in graft mobility. At this point, it is not necessary to redo the graft. Raising a partial thickness flap that includes the graft, removing the loose tissues above the periosteum, and resuturing generally solve the problem.

VARIATION ON THE SAME THEME: FREE CONNECTIVE TISSUE GRAFT

Use of a de-epithelialized graft can increase the amount of attached gingiva (Edel 1974). The gingiva is reported to be stable at 6 months with a mean contraction of 28%. There is complete epithelialization of the connective tissue surface at 2 weeks, with the graft blending into the surrounding tissues at 6 weeks.

FREE GINGIVAL AUTOGRAFT FOR ROOT COVERAGE

Technique

The technique and armamentarium of the free gingival autograft for root coverage are basically the same as the free gingival autograft to increase keratinized tissue with the addition of the steps listed next (Figs. 5.14–5.17).

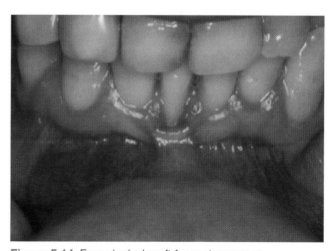
Figure 5.14 Free gingival graft for root coverage.

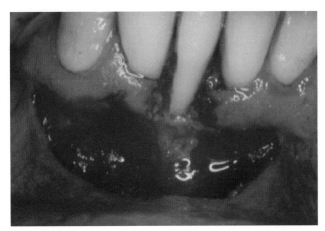

Figure 5.15 A large periosteal bed is prepared to receive the graft. The large size of the bed is to compensate for the avascular area of the root to be covered and eliminate frenum fiber attachment.

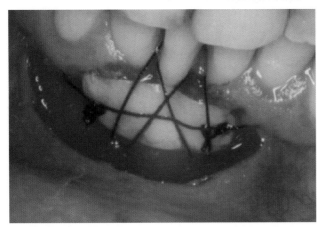

Figure 5.16 The palatal graft is sutured to the recipient bed by using a mesiodistal horizontal suture and two circular intraperiosteal sutures.

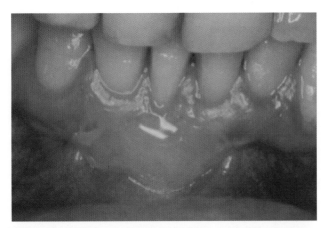

Figure 5.17 The area 1 year later. Take note of the root coverage on tooth 25, the amount of keratinized gingiva, and the absence of labial frenum pull.

Preparation of the Recipient Site

After anesthesia, thorough root planning of the recession by using a Gracey curette or back-action chisel is recommended. This removes the contaminated cementum and flattens the root surface, if necessary. Any concavity or convexity on the root surface should be eliminated or reduced at this stage by using hand or rotary instruments.

Immediately after root planning, saturated citric acid is burnished into the root surface for 5 min by using cotton pellets (Miller 1985). An alternative to citric acid is tetracycline HCl, 50–100 mg/ml, for 3–5 min. This opens the dentinal tubules (Polson et al. 1984) and removes the smear layer that could act as a barrier to the connective tissue attachment to the root surface (Isik et al. 2000). The area is rinsed thoroughly, and horizontal incisions are made at the level of the CEJ, preserving the interdental papillae.

This is followed by vertical incisions at least one tooth away from each side of the recession. This point is critical because the portion of the free gingival graft placed over the denuded root will not survive if there is not a recipient bed large enough to provide collateral vascularization. Therefore, the bed should be as wide as possible, given the anatomical limitation of the area. It should extend apically at least 3 mm below the margin of the denuded root. The wider the bed, the better chance the patient has for root coverage.

Graft Healing

This includes all of the aforementioned steps plus the advent of a creeping attachment, as described by Matter (1980). This phenomenon provides additional root coverage during healing, which may be observed between 1 month and 1 year after grafting. An average of 1.2 mm of coronal creep at 1 year has been reported (Matter 1980).

REFERENCES

Bjorn, H. (1963) Free transplantation of gingival propria. *Svensk Tandlakare Tidskrift* 22, 684–685.

Breault, L.G., Fowler, E.B., & Billman, M.A. (1999) Retained free gingival graft rugae: A 9-year case report. *Journal of Periodontology* 70, 438–440.

Cohen, E.S. (1994) *Atlas of Cosmetic and Reconstructive Periodontal Surgery*. Philadelphia: Lea and Febiger.

Davis, J.S., & Traut, H.F. (1925) Origin and development of the blood supply of whole-thickness skin grafts. *Annals of Surgery* 82, 871–879.

Dordick, B., Coslet, J.G., & Seibert, J.S. (1976) Clinical evaluation of free autogenous gingival grafts placed on alveolar bone. *Journal of Periodontology* 41, 559–567.

Edel, A. (1974) Clinical evaluation of free connective tissue grafts used to increase the width of keratinized tissue. *Journal of Clinical Periodontology* 1, 185–196.

Egli, U., Vollmer, W., & Rateitschak, K.H. (1975) Follow-up studies of free gingival grafts. *Journal of Clinical Periodontology* 2, 98–104.

Ellegaard, B., Karring, T., & Loe, H. (1974) New periodontal attachment procedure based on retardation of epithelial migration. *Journal of Clinical Periodontology* 1, 75–88.

Foman, S. (1960) *Cosmetic Surgery*. Philadelphia: Lippincott.

Holbrook, T., & Ochsenbein, C. (1983) Complete coverage of the denuded root surface with a one stage gingival graft. *International Journal of Periodontics and Restorative Dentistry* 3(3), 9–27.

Hollingshead, W.H. (1968) *The Head and Neck Anatomy for Surgeons*, vol. 1, 2nd edition. Hagerstown, MD: Harper & Row.

Isik, A.G., Tarim, B., Hafez, A.A., Yalcin, F.S., Onan, U., & Cox, C.F. (2000) A comparative scanning electron microscopic study on the characteristics of demineralized dentin root surface using different tetracycline HCl concentrations and application times. *Journal of Periodontology* 71, 219–225.

James, W.C., & McFall, W.T. (1978) Placement of free gingival grafts on denuded alveolar bone. *Journal of Periodontology* 49, 283–290.

Matter, J. (1980) Creeping attachment of free gingival grafts: A 5-year follow-up study. *Journal of Periodontology* 51, 681–685.

Miller, P.D. (1985) Root coverage using the free soft tissue autograft following citric acid application. III. A successful and predictable procedure in areas of deep wide recession. *International Journal of Periodontics and Restorative Dentistry* 5(2), 15–37.

Orban, B.J. (1996) *Oral Histology and Embryology*, 6th edition. Edited by H. Sicher. St. Louis: C.V. Mosby.

Polson, A.M., Frederick, G.T., Ladenheim, S., & Hanes, P.J. (1984) The production of a root surface smear layer by instrumentation and its removal by citric acid. *Journal of Periodontology* 55, 443–446.

Redman, R.S., Shapiro, B.L., & Gonlin, R.J. (1965) Measurement of normal and reportedly malformed palatal vaults. II. Normal juvenile measurements. *Journal of Dental Research* 45, 266–267.

Reese, J.D., & Stark, R.B. (1961) Principles of free skin grafting. *Bulletin of New York Academy of Medicine* (Ser 2) 37, 213.

Reiser, G.M., Bruno, J.F., Mahan, P.E., & Larkin, L.H. (1996) The subepithelial connective tissue graft palatal donor site: Anatomic considerations for surgeons. *International Journal of Periodontics and Restorative Dentistry* 16, 131–137.

Sullivan, H., & Atkins, J. (1968) Free autogenous gingival grafts. I. Principles of successful grafting. *Periodontics* 6, 121–129.

Chapter 6 Subepithelial Connective Tissue Graft

Serge Dibart and Mamdouh Karima

HISTORY

First described in the literature in 1985 (Langer & Langer 1985; Raetzke 1985) as a predictable means for root coverage, a subepithelial connective tissue graft combines the use of a partial thickness flap with the placement of a connective tissue graft. This enables the graft to benefit from a double vascularization, from both the periosteum and the buccal flap.

In addition, the connective tissue carries the genetic message for the overlying epithelium to be keratinized (Edel 1974). Therefore, only connective tissue from a keratinized mucosa should be used as a graft. The partial thickness flap may or may not have vertical releasing incisions (Langer & Langer 1985; Raetzke 1985; Bruno 1994).

Vertical releasing incisions will noticeably reduce the blood supply of the flap. The gingiva is vascularized from the apical area, the interdental septum, and the periosteum. An envelope or a pouch design, without the vertical incisions, has a better likelihood for success than does a flap with vertical releasing incisions. The advantages of the technique are the maintenance of the blood supply to the flap, a close adaptation to the graft, and reduction in postoperative discomfort and scarring.

The predictability and superior aesthetics provided by this technique make it the gold standard for root coverage. Jahnke et al. (1993) reported a success rate fivefold greater for achieving 100% root coverage when using a connective tissue graft versus a thick free gingival graft.

INDICATIONS

- Root coverage in areas of gingival recession (mild, moderate, or severe)
- Gingival coverage of exposed implant abutment or metal collar
- Increase in the width of attached gingiva
- Ridge augmentation (edentulous area)

ARMAMENTARIUM

This includes the basic surgical kit plus citric acid pH 1 (40%) or one capsule of tetracycline hydrochloride (HCl) 250 mg.

TECHNIQUE (ENVELOPE FLAP)

Preparation of the Recipient Site

Root Coverage

After anesthesia, thorough root planning of the recession by using a Gracey curette (Hu-Friedy, Chicago, IL, USA) or back-action chisel is recommended. This will remove the contaminated cementum and flatten the root surface, if necessary. Any concavity or convexity on the root surface should be eliminated or reduced at this stage by using hand or rotary instruments.

Immediately after root planning, saturated citric acid is burnished into the root surface for 5 min by using cotton pellets (Miller 1985). An alternative to citric acid is tetracycline HCl (50–100 mg/ml for 3–5 min). This will open the dentinal tubules (Polson 1984) and remove the smear layer that could act as a barrier to the connective tissue attachment from the root surface (Isik et al. 2000).

Gingival Coverage of an Implant Collar

Clean the metal collar thoroughly by using a cotton pellet soaked with tetracycline HCl (100 mg/ml). There is no need to scale the exposed collar (Fig. 6.1).

Incisions and Creation of the "Pouch"

The technique is similar for root coverage or implant coverage.

The area is rinsed thoroughly and a horizontal incision is made from the cemento-enamel junction (CEJ) to the CEJ on each side of the gingival recession with a no. 15 blade. The blade is then kept almost parallel to the long axis of the tooth, with the blade tip aimed at the underlying bone to keep the buccal flap from perforating.

Practical Periodontal Plastic Surgery, Second Edition. Edited by Serge Dibart.
© 2017 John Wiley & Sons, Inc. Published 2017 by John Wiley & Sons, Inc.

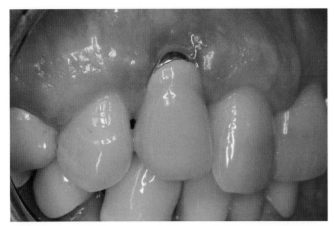

Figure 6.1 The metal collar of the implant showing compromised aesthetics.

A pouch is created through sharp dissection, which has to be carried beyond the mucogingival line to mobilize the buccal flap to reach the CEJ coronally. The pouch is ready when a periodontal probe placed below the recession can coronally move the buccal flap to the CEJ without trouble.

Harvesting the Graft from the Donor Site

Two parallel incisions, perpendicular to the long axis of the teeth, are made in the palate, close to the CEJ (Langer & Langer 1985). Two vertical releasing incisions help dissect the superficial flap and free the subepithelial connective tissue graft (Fig. 6.2). Stay within the safety zone, anterior to the palatal root of the first molar and within 12 mm of the CEJ. Once the graft is harvested, the success rate of the procedure does not appear to be influenced by removing the epithelial collar from the graft (Bouchard et al. 1994).

Suturing of the Graft

The graft is inserted in the subepithelial space created beneath the flap (Fig. 6.3). The coronal portion of the graft lies at, or

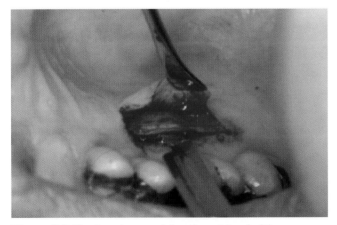

Figure 6.2 The trapdoor enabling the retrieval of the connective tissue graft.

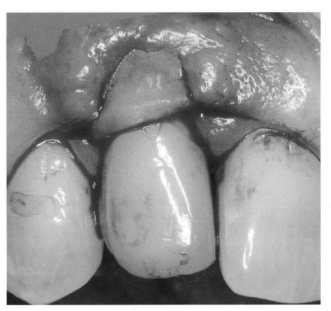

Figure 6.3 The envelope flap (pouch) has been created and the connective tissue graft inserted.

slightly above, the CEJ level, and the graft is secured to the papillae by using resorbable single interrupted sutures. The buccal flap is then pulled upward over the graft with a sling suture (Fig. 6.4). This helps give the graft maximal buccal coverage and ensure optimal vascularization.

It is useful at this stage to insert the curved end of a periosteal elevator (24G or Pritchard) (Hu-Friedy) between the graft and

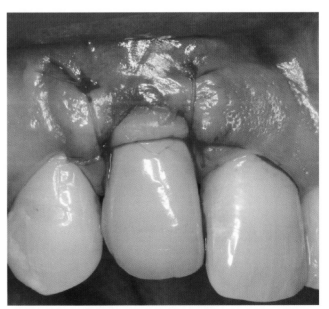

Figure 6.4 The graft is sutured to the papillae, and the buccal flap is sutured over the graft by using a sling suture. It is important to cover as much of the graft as possible to maximize vascular supply.

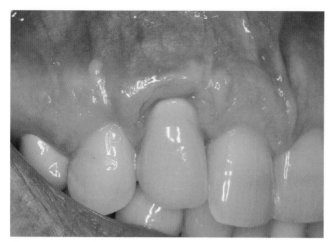

Figure 6.5 After 3 months, the aesthetics have been improved tremendously by the procedure.

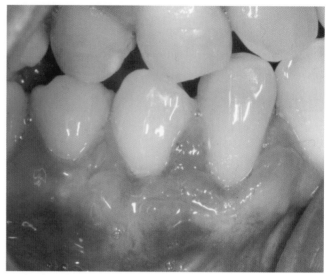

Figure 6.7 Results of 100% root coverage 3 weeks after periodontal microsurgery.

the flap prior to suturing. This will guide the needle when suturing the buccal flap. The needle slides on the elevator and does not engage the graft, enabling the buccal flap to move upward and cover the graft as much as possible. Wet gauze is applied with mild pressure on the wound to minimize dead space between the recipient site, the graft, and the flap. A periodontal dressing is applied on the graft and left for 1 week. The healing is usually uneventful and the results predictable (Figs. 6.5–6.7).

Suturing of the Donor Site

Suture the palatal flap back into position immediately after taking the donor tissue; this will reduce the size of the blood clot, which could cause tissue necrosis. Homeostasis is best accomplished with horizontal mattress sutures in the following way: the sutures (a) pass through a mesial interproximal space on the buccal surface, (b) penetrate the palatal mucosa apical

and distal to the base of the graft site, (c) exit the palate mesially, and (d) cross to the distal interproximal space to be tied on the buccal surface.

This method of suturing compresses the palatal flap, approximates the wound edges (primary intention healing), and provides homeostasis. Since there is no denuded palatal area, the patient reports less postoperative discomfort than with a free gingival graft and less risk of postoperative bleeding. Dressing on the palate is optional.

Possible Complication

Bleeding (please refer to Chapter 5).

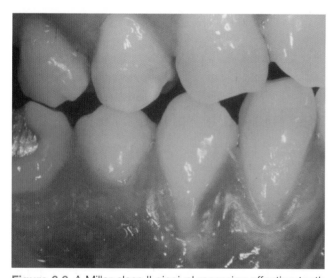

Figure 6.6 A Miller class II gingival recession affecting teeth 27 and 28.

REFERENCES

Bouchard, P., Etienne, D., Ouhayoun, J.P., & Nilveus, R. (1994) Subepithelial connective tissue grafts in the treatment of gingival recessions: A comparative study of two procedures. *Journal of Periodontology* 65, 929–936.

Bruno, J.F. (1994) Connective tissue graft technique assuring wide root coverage. *International Journal of Periodontics and Restorative Dentistry* 14, 127–137.

Edel, A. (1974) Clinical evaluation of free connective tissue grafts used to increase the width of keratinized gingiva. *Journal of Clinical Periodontology* 1, 185–196.

Isik, A.G., Tarim, B., Hafez, A.A., Yalcin, F.S., Onan, U., & Cox, C.F. (2000) A comparative scanning electron microscopic study on the characteristics of demineralized dentin root surface using different tetracycline HCl concentrations and application times. *Journal of Periodontology* 71, 219–225.

Jahnke, P.V., Sandifer, J.B., Gher, M.E., Gray, J.L., & Richardson, A.C. (1993) Thick free gingival and connective tissue autografts for root coverage. *Journal of Periodontology* 64, 315–322.

Langer, B., & Langer, L. (1985) Subepithelial connective tissue graft technique for root coverage. *Journal of Periodontology* 56, 715–720.

Miller, P.D. (1985) Root coverage using the free soft tissue autograft following citric acid application. III. A successful and predictable procedure in areas of deep wide recession. *International Journal of Periodontics and Restorative Dentistry* 5(2), 15–37.

Polson, A.M., Frederick, G.T., Ladenheim, S., & Hanes, P.J. (1984) The production of a root surface smear layer by instrumentation and its removal by citric acid. *Journal of Periodontology* 55, 443–446.

Raetzke, P.B. (1985) Covering localized areas of root exposure employing the "envelope" technique. *Journal of Periodontology* 56, 397–402.

Chapter 7 Pedicle Grafts: Rotational Flaps and Double-Papilla Procedure

Serge Dibart and Mamdouh Karima

HISTORY

Grupe & Warren were the first to describe the sliding flap as a method to repair isolated gingival defects (1956). They reported elevating a full-thickness flap one tooth away from the defect and rotating it to cover the recession. In 1967, Hattler reported the use of a sliding partial thickness flap to correct mucogingival defects on two or three adjacent teeth.

In 1968, Cohen & Ross, using the interproximal papillae to cover recessions and correct gingival defects in areas of insufficient gingiva not suitable for a lateral sliding flap, described the double-papilla repositioned flap. This technique offers the advantages of dual blood supply and denudation of interdental bone only, which is less susceptible to permanent damage after surgical exposure. A full-thickness or partial thickness flap may be used. The latter is preferable because it offers the advantage of quicker healing in the donor site and reduces the risk of facial bone height loss, particularly if the bone is thin or the presence of a dehiscence or a fenestration is suspected (Wood et al. 1972).

Indeed, Wood et al. (1972) reported increased bone at healing time with a partial thickness flap as opposed to a full-thickness flap (0.98 mm versus 0.62 mm). The advantage of the pedicle graft versus the free gingival autograft is the presence of its own blood supply, in the base, that will nourish the graft and facilitate the reestablishment of vascular anastomoses at the recipient site during the healing phase.

INDICATIONS

- Inadequate amount of attached gingiva
- Single or multiple adjacent recessions that have adequate donor tissue laterally (root coverage)
- Recession next to an edentulous area

PREREQUISITES

- Thick periodontal biotype
- Preferably deep vestibule

ARMAMENTARIUM

This includes the basic surgical kit for the lateral sliding and obliquely rotated flaps. For the double papilla, add:

- Tetracycline hydrochloride 250-mg capsule
- Gracey (Hu-Friedy, Chicago, IL, USA) curette no. 1/2
- Scalpel handle mounted with surgical blade no. 15C
- Wide-field surgical loupes (×4.5)
- Titanium instruments for microsurgery:
  - Two straight forceps
  - One straight strong forceps
  - One curved needle holder with lock
  - One straight scissors
- P-1 needle with a 7-0 coated vicryl suture

LATERAL SLIDING FLAP

Technique

After proper anesthesia (Fig. 7.1), the tissue bordering the defect is trimmed free of sulcular epithelium with a blade no. 15 and the root(s) thoroughly planned. When there is enough gingival thickness, a partial thickness flap twice as wide as the defect is reflected beyond the mucogingival junction (Fig. 7.2). The flap is then moved laterally to cover the exposed root, leaving the donor site exposed. The latter is covered by the periosteum/connective tissue (partial thickness flap) or bare bone

Practical Periodontal Plastic Surgery, Second Edition. Edited by Serge Dibart.
© 2017 John Wiley & Sons, Inc. Published 2017 by John Wiley & Sons, Inc.

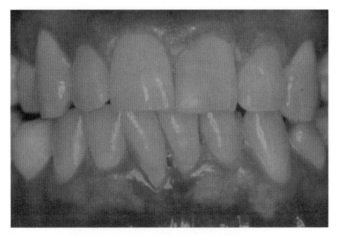

Figure 7.1 Recessions on teeth 24 and 25.

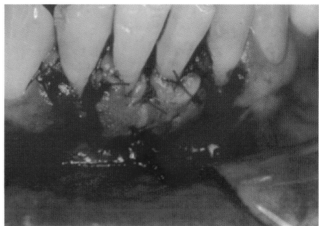

Figure 7.3 The two partial thickness lateral pedicle flaps are sutured covering the exposed root surfaces of teeth 24 and 25.

(full-thickness flap). The flap is then secured using 5-0 single interrupted sutures (Fig. 7.3).

It is sometimes necessary to make a short oblique releasing incision at the base of the flap to avoid any tension that may impair the vascular circulation when the flap is positioned.

This enables the flap to lie flat and firm without excess tension at the base. Pressure is exercised on the flap with fingers and wet gauze to minimize blood clot thickness and encourage fibrinous adhesion. A periodontal dressing is applied on the wound and left in place for 1 week.

A Word of Caution

When operating on the lower mandible in the premolar region, take care not to injure the mental nerve. To avoid this injury, take a preoperative periapical radiograph of the area that will help locate the mental foramen, which is usually located between the first and second premolars, halfway between the alveolar

crest and the lower border of the mandible. Traumatizing or severing the mental nerve can cause temporary or permanent lip and gingival paresthesia. Using a full-thickness flap approach will help minimize this possibility because a blunt dissection is used, and the emergence of the neurovascular bundle from the mental foramen during dissection can be seen.

Wound Healing

The laterally positioned flap will be healing with an attachment to the exposed root (Fig. 7.4). This attachment may be a connective tissue attachment, a long junctional epithelium, or a combination of the two (Wilderman & Wentz 1965). Avoid probing or scaling that area for 6 months. Coverage of the exposed root surfaces with this technique has varied from 60% to 72% (Albano et al. 1969; Smukler 1976; Guinnard & Caffesse 1978).

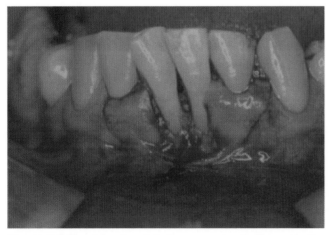

Figure 7.2 Two lateral pedicle flaps are raised adjacent to the receding areas.

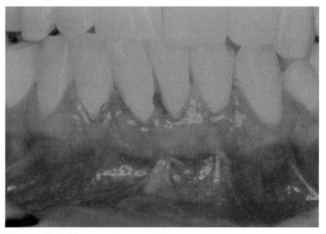

Figure 7.4 The area 1 year later.

Possible Complications

The most common complication is a slight recession at the donor site. This is most likely to occur if the periodontium is thin (thin biotype), with thin gingiva and thin underlying alveolar bone.

Another complication is necrosis or loosening of the flap. This happens if the flap is too thin, in a partial thickness flap, because of faulty technique or inadequate anatomy. The flap will loosen if the dissection was insufficient, and the flap was sutured with tension.

OBLIQUELY ROTATED FLAP

This is a variation of the laterally positioned flap (Pennel et al. 1965). The pedicle is rotated obliquely (90°) and sutured to the underlying connective tissue bed.

DOUBLE-PAPILLA PROCEDURE

Technique

Root Surface Conditioning

Use a Gracey curette no. 1/2 for scaling and root planning to treat the diseased root surface to make it biologically compatible with a healthy periodontium (Jones & O'Leary 1978) (Fig. 7.5). This includes removing the endotoxins, bacteria, and other antigens found in the cementum of the root surface.

Another form of root conditioning is performed by topical application of 50 mg/ml tetracycline for 5 min (Wikesjö et al. 1986). This is accomplished by dissolving the content of a 250-mg

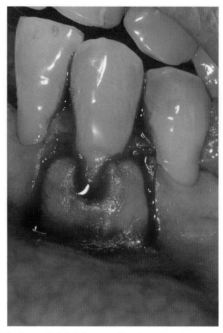

Figure 7.6 A partial thickness flap is raised.

tetracycline capsule in 5 ml saline. Using a Q-tip, apply the tetracycline mix on the root surface and then thoroughly irrigate the root surface with water and dry it with air.

Preparation of the Recipient and Donor Sites

Two horizontal incisions are made on both sides, parallel to the cemento-enamel junction of the tooth to be treated with a no. 15C blade. Vertical incisions are made on the mesial and the distal aspects at the surgical site and placed at the line angles of adjacent teeth (Fig. 7.6). The releasing incision is extended into alveolar mucosa without making contact with the bone.

A scalloped partial thickness internal bevel incision is made in the interdental papilla with a no. 15C blade. A partial thickness pedicle flap with sufficient mesial and distal interdental papilla is prepared. The no. 15C blade is guided to the gingival margin. After the vertical incision is made, the blade should be advanced coronally from the apical of the alveolar mucosa. A partial thickness flap is prepared.

When making the incision, always hold the blade tip parallel to the gingival surface. Undermine the interdental papilla while lifting the papilla gently with the side of the blade. Separate it from the underlying connective tissue. It is important to preserve the mesiodistal width of the interdental papilla on both sides. Use the papilla flap on either end as the donor tissue. Mesially and distally displace the two papilla flaps by half a tooth. The flaps should be wider than the recipient site to cover the root and provide a broad margin for attachment to the connective tissue border around the root.

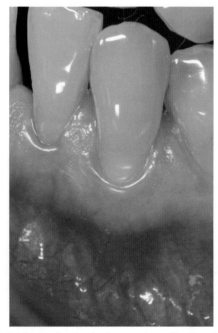

Figure 7.5 Moderate gingival recession affecting the canine.

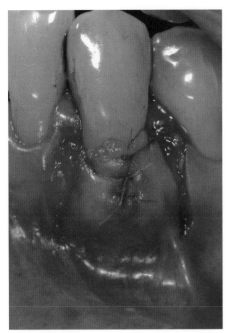

Figure 7.7 The papillae are secured with single interrupted 7.0 sutures.

Suturing Technique

Have the ×4.5 wide-field surgical loupes on before beginning the suturing procedure. Using the microsurgical titanium straight forceps and curved needle holder with lock, suture both papilla flaps at the center of the root surface to ensure coverage of the denuded root surface. Place interrupted sutures (7-0 coated vicryl is preferred) across the medial surface of the two papilla flaps, beginning apically and working coronally. No more than two or three sutures are usually necessary. A sling suture is carried around the tooth and tied facially to prevent the graft from slipping apically (Fig. 7.7).

Apply gentle but firm pressure to the flap for 2–3 min with cotton-free gauze moistened with sterile saline solution to further secure a successful connection. To protect the surgical area during the initial phase of healing, apply a periodontal dressing, which protects the flap from displacement. The dressing must not displace the flap or impinge on its base. An improperly placed dressing may impede the blood supply to the coronal part of the flap and cause necrosis and failure.

At 1 week, the patient is instructed to use a Q-tip dipped in chlorhexidine gluconate in lieu of a toothbrush to cleanse the area. Gentle brushing of the area is initiated 2 months later (Fig. 7.8).

Possible Complications

Few clinical situations would require this procedure because many recession areas are too wide for the papilla. The only complication one might encounter, other than necrosis of the

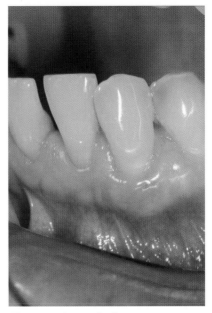

Figure 7.8 The area 2 months later.

flap, is swelling and bruising at the recipient site. This is easily managed with warm pads and anti-inflammatory medications.

Suturing the two flaps over the root surface impairs blood supply, and poor results often occur using this technique. In practice, many clinicians have had limited success with the double-papilla flap. The combination connective tissue graft–double-papilla flap may increase the success rate of the procedure (Nelson 1987).

THE PALATAL "SLIDING" FLAP

First described by Matthews in 2008 as the "pediculated connective tissue graft" this flap is used when large soft tissue defects are present (Figs. 7.9 and 7.10).

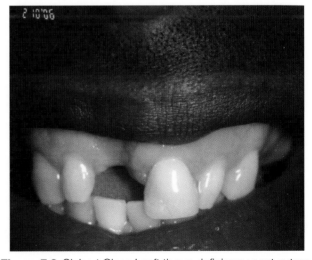

Figure 7.9 Siebert Class I soft tissue deficiency post extraction of tooth 8.

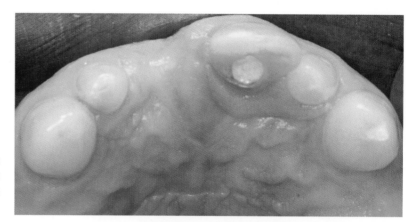

Figure 7.10 Occlusal view showing the buccal-lingual discrepancy. Tooth 9 has a compromised endodontic treatment. It will be extracted later.

The advantage of this flap is the versatility of use to restore horizontal as well as vertical volume loss. This is an essential component of pre-prosthetic implant surgery to achieve superior esthetic results in the maxillary anterior zone.

Technique

After careful infiltration anesthesia on the buccal and palatal sites, a first superficial horizontal incision is made in the palate close to the teeth or the edentulous crest using a scalpel with a no. 15 blade (Fig. 7.11). This first incision has to extend to the recipient site as well. A small distal releasing incision is useful to be able to "flap" the superficial palatal tissue back. Care must be taken to avoid injuring the palatal artery during this process. A periosteal elevator is used to elevate the superficial palatal flap after sharp dissection. A second incision is made into the exposed palatal connective tissue to harvest the palatal pedicle (Fig. 7.12). The mesial attachment of the pedicle must not be severed as it will provide nutrition to the sliding connective tissue graft.

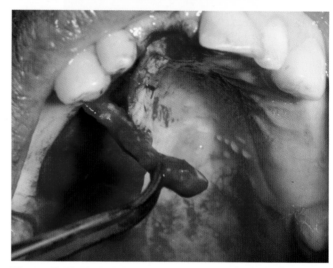

Figure 7.12 The sliding pedicle flap is harvested from within the thickness of the palatal tissue and rotated forward.

The harvested pedicle is held with a surgical tissue plier, rotated on itself and "tucked" under the gingiva of the area with the soft tissue deficiency (Figs 7.13 and 7.14).

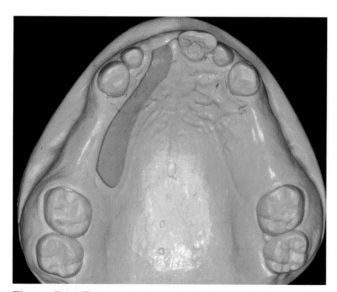

Figure 7.11 The surgical palatal sliding pedicle flap on the patient's plaster model.

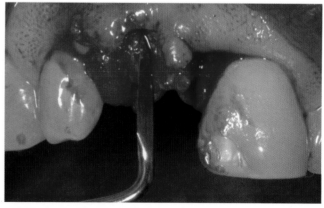

Figure 7.13 The "loose" end of the pedicle flap is tucked buccally under the gingiva.

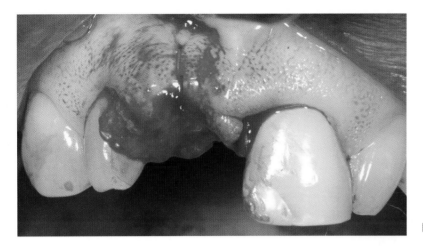

Figure 7.14 The pedicle is sutured bucally.

It is easier to tuck the mesial edge of the pedicle under the periosteum of the gingiva in the area of interest. A single interrupted 5-0 chromic gut suture can be used to secure that edge of the gaft under the buccal gingiva. The suture will anchor the pedicle graft buccally and apically. The rest of the palate can now be sutured with 4-0 or 5-0 chromic gut single interrupted sutures to achieve flap closure and hemostasis.

Six months post surgery the gingival volume is stable enough to place an implant and start the prosthetic reshaping of the site (Figs. 7.15–7.17). Final restoration can be cemented 9 months post soft tissue augmentation surgery (Fig. 7.18).

Possible Complications

Bleeding

Due to the aggressiveness of the procedure bleeding is common. It can be controlled with careful dissection during surgery and the use of a local anesthetic with a 1/50,000 epinephrine

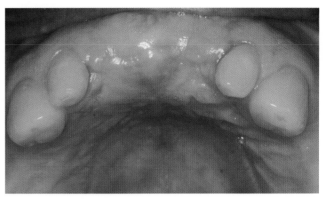

Figure 7.16 Occlusal view showing successful soft tissue volume restoration.

concentration. Using hemostatic resorbable agents placed inside the flap at the time of suturing is also useful to avoid delayed bleeding.

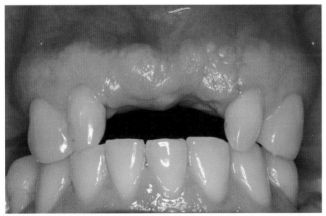

Figure 7.15 Six months post surgery. The gingival volume is restored in a horizontal and vertical dimension. Tooth 9 has been extracted and grafted with bone particulates.

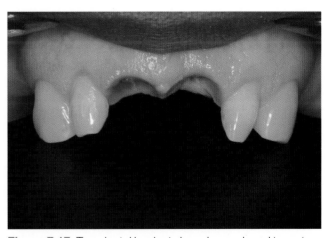

Figure 7.17 Two dental implants have been placed to restore teeth 8 and 9. The provisional restorations have shaped the inter-implant papilla and given a harmonious peri-implant gingival architecture that will complement the final prosthetic crowns.

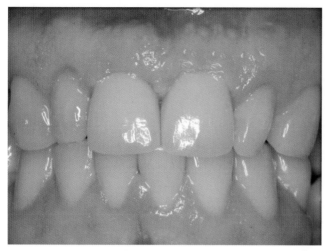

Figure 7.18 Nine months later with the final prosthetic crowns for teeth 8 and 9. Image courtesy of Dr. Adam Ishgi.

Palatal Flap Necrosis

This will happen if the "superficial" palatal flap has been dissected too thinly. Palliative treatment with analgesics and mouth rinses are usually enough to let the wound heal for 2–3 weeks.

REFERENCES

Albano, E.A, Caffessee, R.C., & Carranza, F.A., Jr. (1969) A biometric analysis of laterally displaced pedicle flaps. *Revista de la Asociacion Odontologica Argentina* 57, 351–354.

Cohen, D.W., & Ross, S.E. (1968) The double papilla repositioned flap in periodontal therapy. *Journal of Periodontology* 39, 65–70.

Grupe, H.E., & Warren, R.F. (1956) Repair of gingival defects by a sliding flap operation. *Journal of Periodontology* 27, 92–95.

Guinard, E.A., & Caffesse, R.G. (1978) Treatment of localized gingival recessions. Part I. Lateral sliding flap. *Journal of Periodontology* 49, 351–356.

Hattler, A.B. (1967) Mucogingival surgery: Utilization of interdental gingiva as attached gingiva by surgical displacement. *Periodontics* 5, 126–131.

Jones, W., & O'Leary, T. (1978). The effectiveness of in vivo root planning in removing bacterial endotoxin from the roots of periodontally involved teeth. *Journal of Periodontology* 49, 337–342.

Matthews, D.P. (2008) The pediculated connective tissue graft: a novel approach for the 'blown-out' site in the esthetic zone. *Compendium of Continuing Education in Dentistry* 29(6): 350–352, 354, 356–357.

Nelson, S.W. (1987) The subepithelial connective graft: A bilaminar reconstructive procedure for the coverage of denuded root surfaces. *Journal of Periodontology* 58, 95–102.

Pennel, B.M., Higgason, J.D., Towner, J.D., King, K.O., Fritz, B.D., & Salden, J.F. (1965) Oblique rotated flap. *Journal of Periodontology* 36, 305–309.

Smukler, H. (1976) Laterally positioned mucoperiosteal pedicle grafts in the treatment of denuded roots. *Journal of Periodontology* 47, 590–595.

Wikesjö, U.M.E., Baker, P., Christersson, L., Genco, R.J., Lyall, R.M., Hic, S., DiFlorio, R.M., & Terranova, V.P. (1986) A biomedical approach to periodontal regeneration: Tetracycline treatment conditions dentin surfaces. *Journal of Periodontal Research* 21, 322–329.

Wilderman, M.N., & Wentz, F.M. (1965) Repair of a dentogingival defect with a pedicle flap. *Journal of Periodontology* 35, 218–231.

Wood, D.L., Hoag, F.M., Donnenfeld, O.W., & Rosenfeld, I.D. (1972) Alveolar crest resorption following full and partial thickness flaps. *Journal of Periodontology* 43, 141–144.

Chapter 8 Pedicle Grafts: Coronally Advanced Flaps

Ronaldo B. Santana and Serge Dibart

HISTORY

An advanced flap is moved by sliding the gingival tissues in a single vector toward the defect in the same axis defined by the incisions. Traditional advanced flap designs employed in periodontal plastic surgery include the semilunar repositioned flap, the coronally positioned flap, and variations of these. The semilunar incision was introduced in oral surgery more than a century ago by Partsch (1898, 1899). This incision or variants thereof have been described in mucogingival procedures for root coverage by Harlan (1906), Harvey (1965), Sumner (1969), Marggraf (1985), and Romanos et al. (1993). New modifications to the technique include incision design and suturing (Haghighat 2006), employment of microsurgical procedures for flap manipulation and suturing (Bittencourt et al. 2006, 2007), and use of EDTA (Bittencourt et al. 2007) or enamel matrix derivative (Straumann Emdogain®) for root conditioning. Bernimoulin et al. (1975) first reported the coronally positioned graft, succeeding grafting with a free gingival autograft. This was a two-stage procedure. In the first stage, a free gingival graft was placed apical to the margins of the recession to be treated. The second stage occurred a few months later, when the graft was coronally positioned over the denuded root surfaces. In 1989, Allen and Miller reported the use of a one-stage, coronally positioned flap associated with citric acid root conditioning aimed at correcting shallow marginal recessions (2.5–4.0 mm).

Gingival recession may occur in either a single tooth or, more frequently, in groups of adjacent teeth. The selection of surgical techniques that allow all gingival recession defects to be corrected in a single surgical procedure with the adjacent soft tissues and resulting in adequate soft tissue thickness and color blending of the surgically treated area is the ultimate goal of periodontal plastic surgery. Coronal advancement of the flap is a fundamental, versatile, periodontal surgical procedure that may include most of the above-mentioned treatment objectives, while allowing for combinations with previous or simultaneous soft tissue grafting and/or use of biologically active substances such as growth factors and enamel matrix derivative. The combined long-term track record, simplicity, efficacy, and versatility of this procedure make it the premier technique of choice for root coverage procedures.

INDICATIONS

- Shallow (<4 mm) single or multiple adjacent recessions that have adequate donor tissue apically (root coverage)

PREREQUISITES

- Miller class I gingival recession – single or multiple
- Minimum of 3 mm of keratinized tissue width apical to the recession
- Thick periodontal biotype
- Preferably deep vestibule

ARMAMENTARIUM

This includes the basic surgical kit for periodontal plastic surgery, including:

- Gracey (Hu-Friedy, Chicago, IL, USA) curette no. 1/2
- Scalpel handle mounted with surgical blade no. 15C
- Wide-field surgical loupes (4.5X)
- PrefGel (Straumann, Switzerland)
- Gelfoam (Pharmacia-Upjohn, Kalamazoo, MI, USA) or Surgicel (Johnson & Johnson, New Brunswick, NJ, USA) (for the two-stage procedure)
- PeriAcryl (GluStitch; Delta, BC, Canada) (for the two-stage procedure)

Titanium instruments for microsurgery:

- Two straight forceps
- One straight strong forceps
- One curved needle holder with lock
- One straight scissors
- P-1 needle with a 7-0 coated vicryl suture

SURGICAL TECHNIQUES

Root Preparation

Thorough root planing is performed with hand, rotary, and ultrasonic instruments in all treated sites. A fine-grain finishing bur (Perio-Set, Intensiv S.A., Grancia, Switzerland) is used to remove sharp edges and grooves. After instrumentation, the root surfaces are washed with saline solution to remove any remaining detached fragments from the defect and surgical field. Additional treatments may include root conditioning with tetracycline, EDTA, or enamel matrix derivative.

SEMILUNAR CORONALLY REPOSITIONED FLAP

The semilunar coronally repositioned flap technique (Tarnow 1986, 1994) is a procedure indicated for the treatment of gingival recessions in areas with minimal labial probing depth and adequate band of keratinized gingiva, and is described as a coronally advanced, tensionless, and sutureless flap that does not involve the adjacent papillae, thus preserving the aesthetics (Tarnow 1986, 1994). The procedure has been indicated for the treatment of single and multiple adjacent gingival recession defects. It is believed that this flap design does not shorten the vestibule and results in perfect color blend with adjacent tissues, with a simple, predictable, and fast procedure (Tarnow 1986, 1994). Modifications of the original procedure include new incision design and suturing (Haghighat 2006), employment of microsurgical procedures for flap manipulation and suturing (Bittencourt et al. 2006, 2007), and use of EDTA root conditioning (Bittencourt et al. 2007).

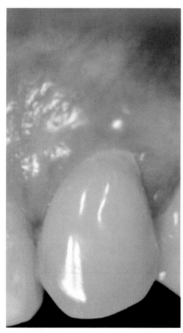

Figure 8.1 Gingival recession on left maxillary canine.

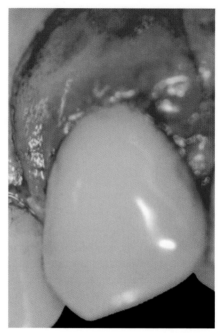

Figure 8.2 Semilunar incision performed. Flap is coronally advanced.

A semilunar incision is carried out following the outline of the gingival margin (Figs. 8.1 and 8.2). This incision end into the papilla on each interproximal area of the tooth to be treated, but not all the way to the tip of the papilla. At least 2 mm of gingiva is preserved on each side of the flap in order to preserve the blood supply (Fig. 8.2). The semilunar incision is curved apically to an extent that guarantees that the apical part of the flap rests on bone after the coronal advancement to cover the root. An intrasulcular incision is performed mid-facially. A split-thickness dissection is then performed from the initial incision coronally to the intrasulcular incision. The mid-facial tissue is completely released, coronally positioned at least 1 mm coronal to the cemento-enamel junction (CEJ) and held in place against the tooth with a moist gauze pad placed with light pressure, perpendicular to the flap, for 5 min. No sutures are placed (Fig. 8.3). The surgical dressing is changed after 7 days and removed after 14 days. A typical outcome is presented in Figs. 8.4 and 8.5

CORONALLY ADVANCED FLAP: SINGLE STAGE

Coronally Repositioned Flap: Restrepo

The flap is made by performing an intrasulcular incision on the buccal/facial aspect of the tooth to be treated. In the interproximal area, the papillae are split in a mesio-distal dimension, resulting in a flat surface of connective tissue for contact between the flap tissues and the retained portion of the papillae after repositioning and suturing of the flap. Two beveled parallel or divergent vertical incisions are then performed in the

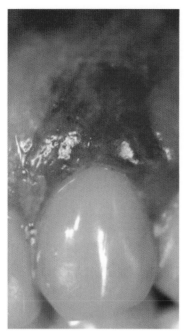

Figure 8.3 One-week healing.

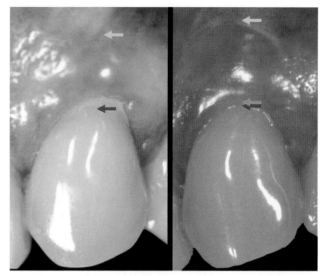

Figure 8.5 Comparison between (a) initial and (b) final aspects. CEJ (blue arrow), gingival margin (green arrow), and muco-gingival junction (yellow arrow).

attached gingiva and continued several millimeters apically into the alveolar mucosa. One incision is placed on the distal aspect of the tooth anterior to the recession being treated and another on the mesial aspect of the tooth distal to the recession. A combined mucoperiosteal–mucosal rectangular or trapezoidal flap is then elevated such that the first 3–4 mm of the coronal aspect of the alveolar bone is exposed, while the remaining buccal bone is still covered by the periosteum and gingival connective tissue. A complementary horizontal incision is performed on the apical aspect of the flap, by means of partial-thickness dissection, releasing the flap from the attached periosteum and muscle fibers. This allows the elongation and free coronal positioning of the flap. Roots are carefully prepared as described above. The flap is then positioned at least 1 mm coronal to the CEJ and maintained in place by means of individual sutures (Figs. 8.6–8.8). A typical clinical outcome is shown in Fig. 8.9

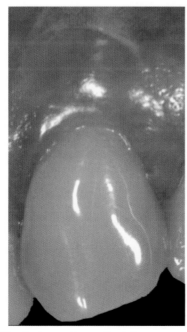

Figure 8.4 Treated area 6 months later.

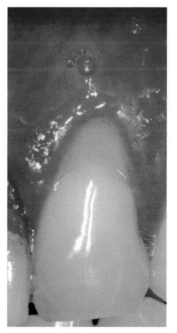

Figure 8.6 Gingival recession on left maxillary canine.

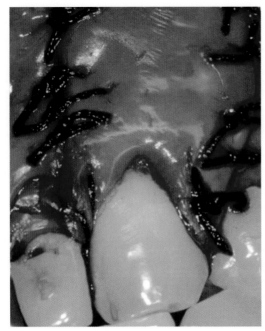

Figure 8.7 Flap is coronally positioned.

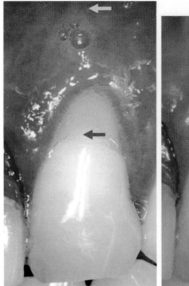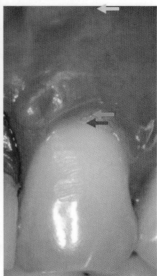

Figure 8.9 Comparison between (a) initial and (b) final aspects. CEJ (blue arrow), gingival margin (green arrow), and muco-gingival junction (yellow arrow).

mesial and distal line angles of the tooth, avoiding the formation of butt joints between the flap and adjacent tissues, and are continued several millimeters apically into the alveolar mucosa (Fig. 8.14).

The vertical incisions are joined by an intrasulcular incision (Fig. 8.12). A combined mucoperiosteal–mucosal trapezoidal flap is elevated such that the first 3-4 mm of the coronal aspect

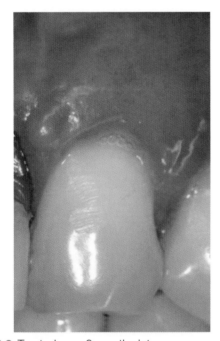

Figure 8.8 Treated area 6 months later.

Coronally Advanced Flap (Allen & Miller 1989)

The flap is designed by making two vertical releasing incisions at the mesial and distal aspects of the recession to be treated, in such a way that neither of the proximal papillae are included as part of the flap (Figs. 8.10–8.13). Papillae are never bisected. Beveled divergent vertical incisions are performed in the attached gingiva, initiating at the CEJ level on the

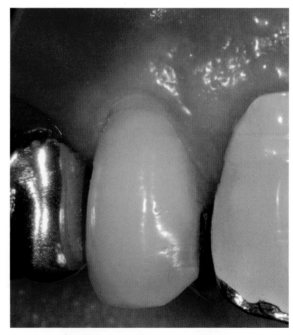

Figure 8.10 Gingival recession is present on maxillary right second molar.

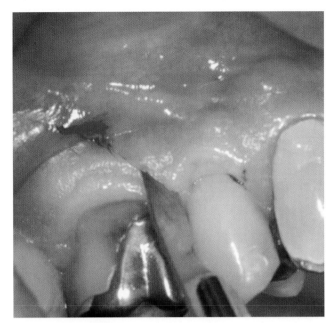

Figure 8.11 Beveled vertical releasing incision on distal aspect of the recession.

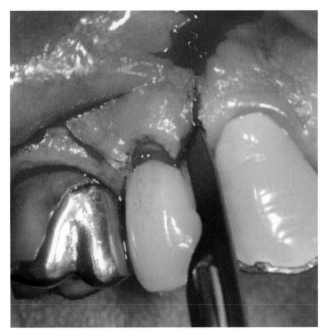

Figure 8.13 Beveled vertical releasing incision on mesial aspect of the recession.

of the alveolar bone is exposed, while the remaining buccal bone is still covered by the periosteum and gingival connective tissue (Figs. 8.15 and 8.16). In the interproximal area, the papillae are split in a mesio-distal dimension, resulting in a flat surface of connective tissue for contact between the flap tissues and the retained portion of the papillae after repositioning and suturing of the flap (Fig. 8.17). A complementary horizontal incision is performed on the apical aspect of the flap,

by means of partial-thickness dissection, releasing the flap from the attached periosteum and muscle fibers. This allows the elongation and free coronal positioning of the flap (Fig. 8.18). Roots are prepared as described above. The flap is then positioned at least 1 mm coronal to the CEJ and maintained in place by means of individual sutures (Fig. 8.19). A typical clinical outcome is shown in Figs. 8.20 and 8.21.

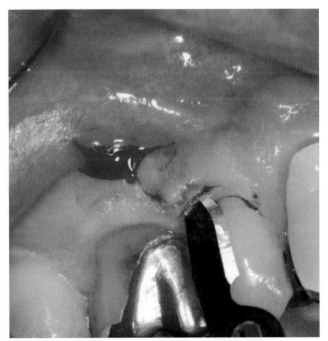

Figure 8.12 Sulcular incision on buccal aspect of the recession.

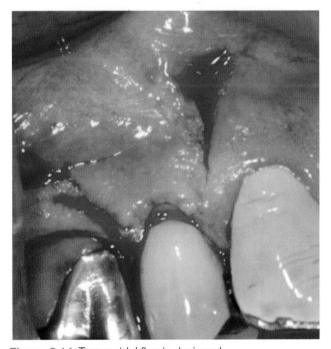

Figure 8.14 Trapezoidal flap is designed.

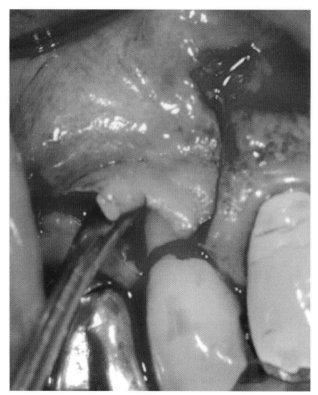

Figure 8.15 Coronal portion of the flap is raised as full thickness.

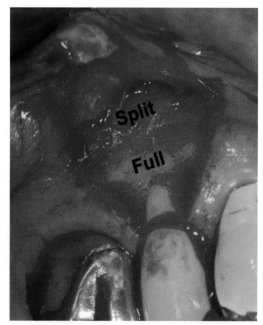

Figure 8.16 A split-thickness dissection is performed in the apical aspect of the flap.

Envelope Technique (Zucchelli & de Sanctis 2000)

The coronally advanced flap procedure is designed as a split–full–split thickness envelope flap (Figs. 8.22–8.26). A

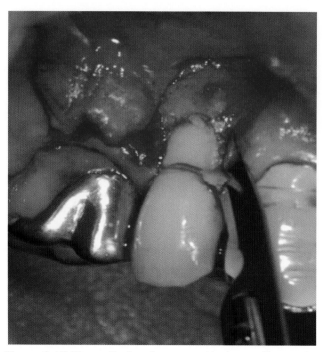

Figure 8.17 The epithelium is removed in the papillary region via split-thickness dissection.

horizontal incision consisting of oblique submarginal incisions is performed in the interdental areas, at both the mesial and distal aspects of the recession to be treated, then joined in an intrasulcular incision at the recession defects. The papillary portion located coronally to the oblique interdental incisions is de-epithelized, while the papillary portion located apically to the oblique incision is split in a mesio-distal dimension, resulting

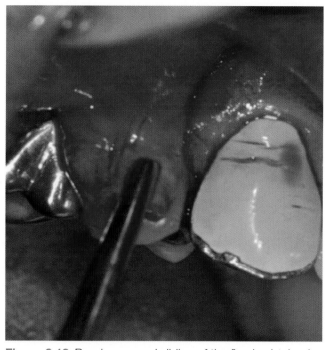

Figure 8.18 Passive coronal sliding of the flap is obtained.

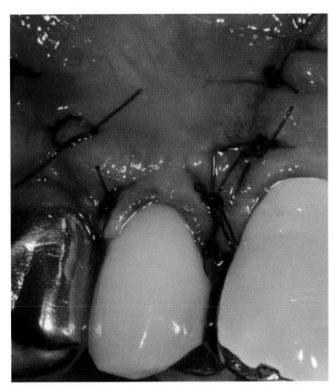

Figure 8.19 Flap is sutured 1–2 mm coronal to the CEJ.

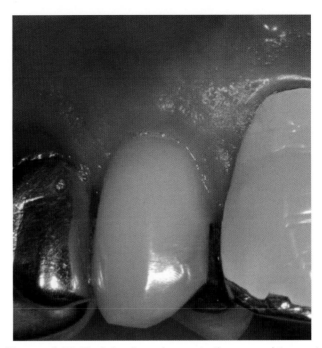

Figure 8.20 Final healing demonstrating complete root coverage.

in a flat surface of connective tissue for contact between the flap tissues and the retained portion of the papillae after repositioning and suturing of the flap. A combined mucoperiosteal–mucosal envelope flap is elevated such that the first 3–4 mm of the coronal aspect of the alveolar bone is exposed, while the remaining buccal bone is still covered by the periosteum and

gingival connective tissue (Fig. 8.23). A complementary horizontal incision is performed on the apical aspect of the flap, by means of partial-thickness dissection, releasing the flap from the attached periosteum and muscle fibers. This allows the elongation and free coronal positioning of the flap. Roots were prepared as described above. The flap is then positioned at least 1 mm coronal to the CEJ and maintained in place by

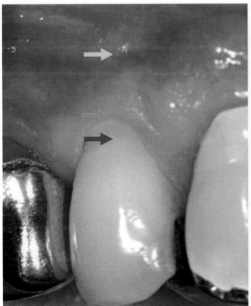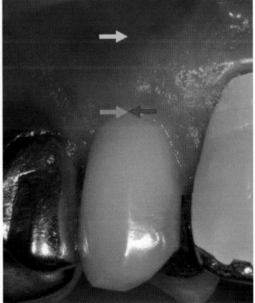

Figure 8.21 Comparison between (a) initial and (b) final aspects. CEJ (blue arrow), gingival margin (green arrow), and mucogingival junction (yellow arrow).

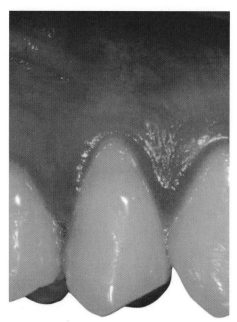

Figure 8.22 Gingival recession is observed on maxillary right first premolar.

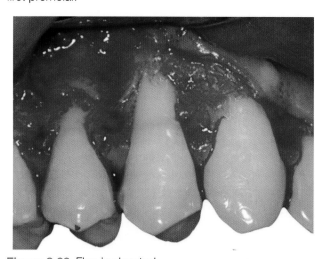

Figure 8.23 Flap is elevated.

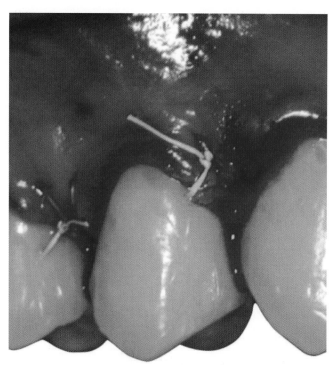

Figure 8.24 Flap is sutured 1–2 mm coronally to the CEJ.

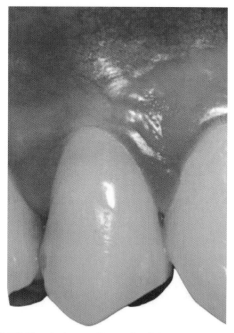

Figure 8.25 Treated area 6 months later.

means of individual monofilament sutures (Fig. 8.24). A typical clinical outcome is shown in Fig. 8.26.

CORONALLY POSITIONED FLAP: TWO STAGES

Technique

First Stage

The first part of a two-stage, coronally positioned flap is a free gingival autograft (see Chapter 5).

Second Stage

After a minimum of 3 months of healing, the gingival graft is coronally positioned to cover the root, which should be carefully

planned and conditioned with citric acid or tetracycline HCl (50–100 mg/ml) for 3–5 min. If the root has a prominent concavity or convexity, it should be eliminated or reduced with a back-action chisel or a burr to graft on a flat surface.

The second stage requires a split-thickness dissection with mesial and distal vertical releasing incisions (Fig. 8.27). The

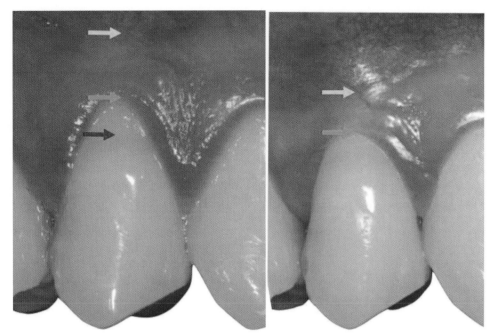

Figure 8.26 Comparison between (a) initial and (b) final aspects. CEJ (blue arrow), gingival margin (green arrow), and muco-gingival junction (yellow arrow).

vertical incisions are made at the line angles of the adjacent teeth when there is a full dentition and are coronally set. The partial thickness pedicle flap, staying close to the periosteum, is then dissected with the scalpel oriented toward the alveolar bone. This will ensure that the flap is not punctured.

The result from this sharp dissection is a very mobile flap that can easily be moved coronally. This mobility is achieved by carrying the dissection beyond the mucogingival junction. The papillae adjacent to the recession are then de-epithelialized with a new no. 15C blade and the flap sutured 0.5–1.0 mm coronal to the CEJ. This is achieved using single interrupted sutures to secure the papilla areas and the vertical releasing incisions (Fig. 8.27). The area is covered with a periodontal dressing and left to heal for 1 week. After 2 months (Fig. 8.28), the patient can start gently brushing the area.

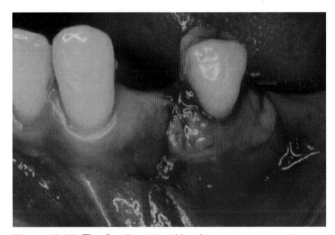

Figure 8.27 The flap is sutured in place.

Post-Surgical Care

Irrespective of the technical variation employed, post-surgical care is performed as previously described (Santana et al. 2010a & b). The surgical dressing (CoePak, USA) is changed after 7 days and removed after 14 days. The patients are put on systemic analgesics consisting of 750 mg of paracetamol every 6 hours for 4 days. The patients are instructed to continue their regular home hygiene care except in the operated area, in which tooth-brushing is discontinued for the first 30 days after surgery and plaque control is maintained by means of gentle topical applications of chlorhexidine gluconate (2.0%) in saturated cotton swabs twice a day. Gentle

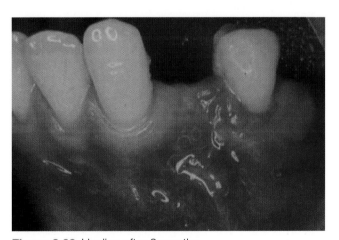

Figure 8.28 Healing after 2 months.

tooth-brushing with an extra-soft-bristle toothbrush is then initiated. Analgesics are prescribed on an individual basis. The sutures are removed 2 weeks after surgery.

Maintenance Schedule

A careful maintenance schedule is essential for optimum results and is performed as previously described (Santana et al. 2010a & b). Following surgery, patients are seen weekly during the first 3 months and bi-weekly for the next 3 months. Maintenance visits consist of reinforcement of oral hygiene procedures and professional supra-gingival coronal polishing. Additional oral chemical plaque control is performed once every 3 months by means of mouth rinses with a solution of chlorhexidine gluconate 0.12% BID, for 1 week.

Wound Healing: Coronally Advanced Flap

The clinical aspects of wound healing following the use of advanced flap in root coverage procedures have been described (Santana et al. 2010a & b). Healing of the coronally advanced flap progressed as normal healing of periodontal flap procedures (Figs. 8.9, 8.21, and 8.26). After 1 week, the wound exhibited minimal color alteration, with reduced edema and erythema. The vertical incisions are clearly distinguishable. These characteristics progressively disappear throughout the 6-month healing period in which the gingival color, texture and contour of the areas treated by the coronally advanced flap procedure appeared essentially identical to the adjacent soft tissues (Figures 8.9, 8.21, and 8.26). Minimal scarring is noticeable in the alveolar mucosa in a minority of sites.

In a recent systematic review on the effects of coronally advanced flap procedures on the treatment of gingival recession defects, Cairo et al. (2008) concluded that the technique resulted in mean gingival recession reduction and complete root coverage. Mean root coverage after the coronally advanced flap procedure varies between 60% and 99% of the previously exposed root surfaces, while complete root coverage could be obtained in 61% to 95% of sites treated in the short term (Allen & Miller 1989; Harris & Harris 1994; Lins et al. 2003; Cortes et al. 2004; da Silva et al. 2004; Huang et al. 2005a & 2005b; Santamaria et al. 2008, 2009; Santana et al. 2010a & b). Lower degrees of root coverage were reported by other authors in long-term studies. Gürgan et al. (2004) reported a mean root coverage of 68.3% after 12 months and 44.9% after 60 months following the coronally advanced flap procedure.

In order to optimize the long-term clinical results following the use of advanced flap in root coverage procedures, the combination of the coronally advanced flap with either a connective tissue graft or enamel matrix derivative is suggested.

Wound Healing: Semilunar Coronally Repositioned Flap

Clinical inspection revealed that areas treated with the semilunar coronally repositioned flap procedure exhibit a distinct aspect of healing pattern (Santana et al. 2010a). In the first week, the flap tissues appear extremely red in color and swollen (Fig. 8.3). In the area of the semilunar incision a white-colored area of debris, resembling a fibrin clot, is frequently found. The wound edges are frequently elevated in relation to the central periosteal region. These aspects persisted, but progressively diminished, during the healing period (Fig. 8.4). The erythemathous aspect may persist for up to 3 months, while the area of the white-colored debris progressively epithelizes in about 2 weeks, but color and texture may remain altered for several months after surgery. A notable semi-lunar white scar is generally present in all the sites treated by the semilunar coronally repositioned flap procedure even several years after the surgical procedure (Figs. 8.4 and 8.5). Thus, this significantly delayed reddish healing phase, followed by a noticeable semilunar white scar located just a few millimeters apical to the CEJ, is a potential drawback for the procedure, especially in patients with a high smile line.

Mean coverage of the exposed root surfaces with this technique has varied from 42% to 91%, while complete root coverage has varied between 9% and 53% (Romanos et al. 1993; Bittencourt et al. 2006; Santana et al. 2010a). Such important discrepancies are likely explained by the differences in the surgical protocols since some authors used additional methods of flap fixation such as sutures (Romanos et al. 1993) or adhesives (Bittencourt et al. 2006, 2007), as well as microsurgical techniques that might have improved the handling of thin and delicate soft tissues during the semilunar coronally repositioned flap procedure (Bittencourt et al. 2006).

The reasons for such sharp differences between the semilunar coronally repositioned flap and coronally advanced flap procedures have been speculated on (Santana et al. 2010b) and are possibly explained by the direction of releasing incisions, the positioning, and the fixation of the flap. In the semilunar coronally repositioned flap, a horizontal incision is performed perpendicular to the axis of the flap movement and parallel to the gingival margin, which is positioned coronally to cover the root surface. This incision may significantly disrupt the vascular supply of the flap, as evidenced by the significantly increased erithema in the surgical site. Moreover, during healing a significant hypertrophic scar is also noted at the area of this incision. The wound contraction that occurs at the base of the flap may pull the flap margin apically, and since no sutures are used to anchor or stabilize the pedicle, there is no antagonistic force in effect to counterpart this action, thus the net result is the apical traction of the flap margin, clinically detected as gingival recession following the semilunar coronally repositioned flap (Petroll et al. 1998). The coronally advanced flap procedure, however, appears to be more stable due to the fact that the releasing incisions are performed parallel to the axis of flap movement, and additional stabilization is obtained by sutures during the critical early healing events (Wikesjö 1992; Werfully et al. 2002), therefore the contraction forces do not act contrary to the axis of tissue displacement.

Moreover, the gingival margin is easily positioned and maintained 1 mm or more coronally to the CEJ in sites treated by the coronally advanced flap procedure. Coronal positioning and stabilization are more critical in sites treated by the semilunar coronally repositioned flap and the use of surgical dressing as the single method for flap stabilization may not be adequate or, at worst, may dislodge the flap during the placement of the dressing. This fact may also impact the results, since the placement and stabilization of the flap coronally to the CEJ is positively correlated with the degree of root coverage following coronally advanced flap.

Possible Complications

The most common complication is lack of complete root coverage. This is most likely to occur if the flap is thinner than 1 mm (Hwang et al. 2005a), in patients with thin gingival biotype (Saletta et al. 2001; Berlucchi et al. 2005), if the flap is not sutured at least 1–2 mm coronal to the CEJ (Pini Prato et al. 2005), if adjacent papillae width and height are reduced (Saletta et al. 2001; Berlucchi et al. 2005), and in the case of lack of control of a traumatic tooth brushing technique (Zucchelli & Wennstrom 1996) or if the patient is a smoker (Chambrone et al. 2009). Another complication of the procedure is necrosis of the flap margins, which will occur if the partial thickness flap is too thin. This, in turn, could result in exposure of the underlying root surface and make an existing recession worse. Partial thickness flaps are not indicated in areas of thin connective tissue. The gingival recession may also recur after a few years.

REFERENCES

Allen, E.P., & Miller Jr, P.D. (1989) Coronal positioning of existing gingiva: short term results in the treatment of shallow marginal tissue recession. *Journal of Periodontology* 60, 316–319.

Berlucchi, I., Francetti, L., Del Fabbro, M., Basso, M., & Weinstein, R.L. (2005) The influence of anatomical features on the outcome of gingival recessions treated with coronally advanced flap and enamel matrix derivative: a 1-year prospective study. *Journal of Periodontology* 76, 899–907.

Bernimoulin, J.P., Luscher, B., & Muhlemann, H. (1975) Coronally repositioned periodontal flap. *Journal of Clinical Periodontology* 2, 1–13.

Bittencourt, S., Ribeiro, E.D.P., Sallum, E.A., Sallum, A.W., Nociti Jr., F.H., & Casati, M.Z. (2006) Comparative 6-month clinical study of a semilunar coronally positioned flap and subepithelial connective tissue graft for the treatment of gingival recession. *Journal of Periodontology* 77, 174–181.

Bittencourt, S., del Peloso Ribeiro, E., Sallum, E.A., Sallum, A., Nociti Jr, F.H., & Casati, M.Z. (2007) Root surface biomodification with EDTA for the treatment of gingival recession with a semilunar coronally repositioned flap. *Journal of Periodontology* 78, 1695–1701.

Cairo, F., Pagliaro, U., & Nieri, M. (2008) Treatment of gingival recession with coronally advanced flap procedures: a systematic review. *Journal of Clinical Periodontology* 35(8), 136–162.

Chambrone, L., Chambrone, D., Pustiglioni, F.E., Chambrone, L.A., & Lima, L.A. (2009) The influence of tobacco smoking on the outcomes achieved by root-coverage procedures: a systematic review. *Journal of the American Dental Association* 140(3), 294–306.

Cortes, A.Q., Martins, A.G., Nociti Jr, F.H., Salllum, A.W., Casati, M.Z., & Sallum, E.A. (2004) Coronally positioned flap with or without acellular dermal matrix graft in the treatment of class I gingival recessions: a randomized controlled clinical study. *Journal of Periodontology* 75, 1137–1144.

da Silva, R.C., Joly, J.C., de Lima, A.F., & Tatakis, D.N. (2004) Root coverage using the coronally positioned flap with or without a subepithelial connective tissue graft. *Journal of Periodontology* 75, 413–419.

Gürgan, C.A., Oruç, A.M., & Akkaya, M. (2004) Alterations in location of the mucogingival junction 5 years after coronally repositioned flap surgery. *Journal of Periodontology* 75, 893–901.

Haghighat, K. (2006) Modified semilunar coronally advanced flap. *Journal of Periodontology* 77, 1274–1279.

Harlan, A.W. (1906) Restoration of gum tissue on the labial aspect of teeth. *Dental Cosmos* 48, 927–928.

Harris, R.J., & Harris, A.W. (1994) The coronally positioned pedicle graft with inlaid margins: a predictable method of obtaining root coverage of shallow defects. *International Journal of Periodontics and Restorative Dentistry* 14, 229–241.

Harvey, P.M. (1965) Management of advanced periodontitis. (I) Preliminary report of a method of surgical reconstruction. *New Zealand Dental Journal* 61, 180–187.

Huang, L.H., Neiva, R.E.F., & Wang, H.L. (2005a) Factors affecting the outcomes of coronally advanced flap root coverage procedure. *Journal of Periodontology* 76, 1729–1734.

Huang, L.H., Neiva, R.E.F., Soehren, S.E., Giannobile, W.V., & Wang, H.L. (2005b) The effect of platelet rich plasma on the coronally advanced flap root coverage procedure: a pilot human trial. *Journal of Periodontology* 76, 1768–1777.

Lins, L.H., de Lima, A.F., & Sallum, A.W. (2003) Root coverage: comparison of coronally positioned flap with or without titanium-reinforced barrier membrane. *Journal of Periodontology* 74, 168–174.

Partsch, C. (1898) Ueber Wurzelresection. *Dtsch Monatsschr Zahnheilkd* 16, 80–86.

Partsch, C. (1899) Ueber Wurzelresection. *Dtsch Monatsschr Zahnheilkd* 17, 348–367.

Petroll, W.M., Cavanagh, H.D., & Jester, J.V. (1998) Assessment of stress fiber orientation during healing of radial keratotomy wounds using confocal microscopy. *Scanning* 20(2), 74–82.

Pini Prato, G.P., Baldi, C., Nieri, M., Franseschi, D., Cortellini, P., Clauser, C., Rotun- do, R., & Muzzi, L. (2005) Coronally advanced flap: the post-surgical position of the gingival margin is an important factor for achieving complete root coverage. *Journal of Periodontology* 76, 713–722.

Romanos, G.E., Bernimoulin, J.P., & Marggraf, E. (1993) The double lateral bridging flap for coverage of denuded root surface: longitudinal study and clinical evaluation after 5 to 8 years. *Journal of Periodontology* 64, 683–688.

Saletta, D., Pini Prato, G., Pagliaro, U., Baldi, C., Mauri, M., & Nieri, M. (2001) Coronally advanced flap procedure: is the interdental papilla a prognostic factor for root coverage? *Journal of Periodontology* 72(6), 760–766.

Santamaria, M.P., Suaid, F.F., Casati, M.Z., Nociti, F.H., Sallum, A.W., & Sallum, E.A. (2008) Coronally positioned flap plus resin-modified glass ionomer restoration for the treatment of gingival recession associated with non-carious cervical lesions: a randomized controlled clinical trial. *Journal of Clinical Periodontology* 79(4), 621–628.

Santamaria, M.P., da Silva Feitosa, D., Nociti Jr, F.H., Casati, M.Z., Sallum, A.W., & Sallum, E.A. (2009) Cervical restoration and the amount of soft tissue coverage achieved by coronally advanced flap: a 2-year follow-up randomized-controlled clinical trial. *Journal of Clinical Periodontology* 36(5), 434–441.

Santana, R.B., Furtado, M.B., Mattos, C.M.L., Fonseca, E.M., & Dibart, S. (2010a) Clinical evaluation of single-stage advanced versus rotated flaps in the treatment of gingival recessions. *Journal of Periodontology* 81, 485–492.

Santana, R.B., Mattos, C.M.L., & Dibart, S. (2010b) A clinical comparison of two flap designs for coronal advancement of the gingival margin: semilunar versus coronally advanced flap. *Journal of Clinical Periodontology* 37, 651–658.

Sumner, C.F. (1969) Surgical repair of recession on the maxillary cuspid: incisally repositioning the gingival tissues. *Journal of Periodontology* 40, 119–121.

Tarnow, D.P. (1986) Semilunar coronally repositioned flap. *Journal of Clinical Periodontology* 13, 182–185.

Tarnow, D.P. (1994) Solving restorative esthetic dilemmas with the semilunar coronally positioned flap. *Journal of Esthetic Dentistry* 6, 61–64.

Werfully, S., Areibi, G., Toner, M., Bergquist, J., Walker, J., Renvert, S., & Claffey, N. (2002) Tensile strength, histological and immunohistochemical observations of periodontal wound healing in the dog. *Journal of Periodontal Research* 37(5), 366–374.

Wikesjö, U.M., Nilvéus, R.E., & Selvig, K.A. (1992) Significance of early healing events on periodontal repair: a review. *Journal Periodontology* 63, 158–165.

Zucchelli, G., & de Sanctis, M. (2000) Treatment of multiple recession-type defects in patients with esthetic demands. *Journal of Periodontology* 71, 1506–1514.

Zucchelli, G., & Wennstrom, J.L. (1996) Increased gingival dimensions. A significant factor for successful outcome of root cover- age procedures? A 2-year prospective clinical study. *Journal of Clinical Periodontology* 23, 770–777.

Chapter 9 Aesthetic and Morphometric Evaluation of the Periodontium

Ronaldo B. Santana

INTRODUCTION

The appearance of the gingival tissues surrounding the teeth plays an important role in the aesthetics of the anterior maxillary region of the mouth since the dento-gingival aesthetics is defined by the labial perimeter and includes teeth, lips, and gingiva. Ideal aesthetics involves the establishment of correct anatomical relationships between the dento-gingival area shown during smiling.

Abnormalities in symmetry and contour can significantly affect the harmonious appearance of the natural or prosthetically restored dentition. Consequently, any dental procedure performed in this zone can be an aesthetic challenge due to the visibility of the dento-gingival interface (Silvestri 2002). Knowledge of external anatomy is a critical element in modern clinical periodontology, allowing clinical decisions regarding diagnosis, treatment, and prognosis to be taken based on specific anatomic relationships. The understanding of the aesthetic anatomic relationships of the gingival tissues has evolved to a treatment concept named geometric gingival anatomic rehabilitation (GEAR), which may allow for trans-disciplinary aesthetic treatment planning in oral rehabilitation based on re-establishment of the ideal parameters of gingival health, function, and aesthetics.

GINGIVAL TOPOGRAPHY

The understanding of the ideal gingival topography has critical importance for multidisciplinary diagnosis and treatment in the anterior dentition. The physiologic gingival architecture has been described as "one in which the interdental area is conical and coronally positioned to the buccal and lingual (or palatal) plates of bone, which have a parabolic shape and flow smoothly from the interdental area; an interdental area that follows the shape of the cementoenamel junction" (Prichard 1961), "allowing a thin, scalloped, knife-edged gingival contour with pyramid-shaped papillae that fill the interproximal space" (Bensimon 1999). This knife-edged, festooned marginal gingival contour is primarily affected by the degree of concavity and convexity of the tooth surface (Grant et al. 1988). Thus, the higher the convexity of the root surface, the more markedly scalloped is the gingival margin.

GINGIVAL CONTOUR

The physiologic gingival architecture has been traditionally described as having a scalloped contour (Prichard 1961; Melcher & Bowen 1969; Schroeder 1986) around the four surfaces of the tooth in accordance with the course of the cementum-enamel junction (Löe et al. 1990; Schroeder 1991) and therefore concave apically in the free surfaces and convex occlusally at the tip of the papilla (Löe et al. 1990). The gingival architecture is defined by the position of the gingival zenith apically and the tip of the interdental papillae coronally (Fig. 9.1).

GINGIVAL ZENITH

The zenith is defined as the apical point of the gingival marginal scallop (Figs. 9.1–9.4). This important anatomic landmark has been described to have a specific spatial orientation in both the apico-coronal and mesio-distal directions (Mattos & Santana 2008). Correct spatial positioning of the zenith following therapeutic manipulation is mandatory, since it can greatly influence the emergence profile and axial inclination of the teeth by modifying the line angle position of the long axis of the emergence of the crown from the gingiva (Mattos & Santana 2008) and thus add the proper symmetry to the entire soft tissue system (Smallwood 2003).

A study has evaluated the position of the gingival zenith in the maxillary anterior dentition in young adults. The gingival topography of the maxillary incisors and canines was measured for the mesio-distal displacement of the gingival zenith in relation to the long axis of the crowns and determining the corono-apical position of the gingival margin of the lateral incisors in relation to the central incisors and canines (Mattos & Santana 2008). The goal was to quantify the spatial relationships of the gingival zenith as an aid for ideal design of marginal gingival positioning following restorative, orthodontic, and periodontal therapy.

Practical Periodontal Plastic Surgery, Second Edition. Edited by Serge Dibart.
© 2017 John Wiley & Sons, Inc. Published 2017 by John Wiley & Sons, Inc.

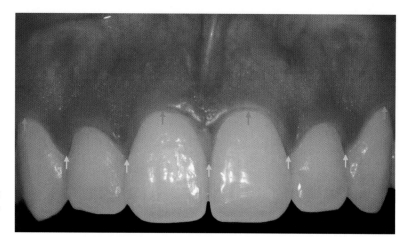

Figure 9.1 Gingival contour. Gingival zenith (green arrows) and interdental papillae (yellow arrows).

LATERAL DISPLACEMENT OF THE GINGIVAL ZENITH

The distal displacement of the zenith is not a universal finding in the anterior maxillary anterior sextant, as previously believed (Stein 1977; Kay 1982; Magne & Belser 2002; Morr 2004). Distinct distributions of displacement were observed for the three groups of teeth studied (Fig. 9.2). Mesial displacement of the zenith in relation to the long axis of the crown was not observed in any tooth, regardless of the tooth group (Fig. 9.2). The distal positioning of the zenith was very frequent in the central incisors, frequent in the lateral incisors, and rare in the canines. In addition, lateral displacement of the zenith was larger in the central incisors than in the lateral incisors, and larger in the lateral incisors than in the canines. In other words, the more anterior the tooth, the higher the prevalence and the bigger the distal displacement of the gingival zeniths (Fig. 9.2).

Contra-lateral comparisons did not reveal significant differences between the tooth groups, thus demonstrating contralateral symmetry for both the distal displacement of the gingival margin and the apical displacement of the zenith of the lateral incisor, a concept agreed by most authors (Stein 1977; Kay 1982; Allen 1988; Rufenacht 1990; Borghetti & Monnet-Corti 2002; Magne & Belser 2002; Morr 2004). The direct quantitative measurements and qualitative descriptive statistics of the relative position of the gingival zenith in the maxillary anterior sextant provide new insights into the anatomic relationships of the gingival margin, with potential clinical applications in the diagnosis and treatment of the gingival complex morphology. These data can be employed clinically to determine the ideal unilateral position of the gingival margin during periodontal, orthodontic, restorative, and orthognatic surgical therapy.

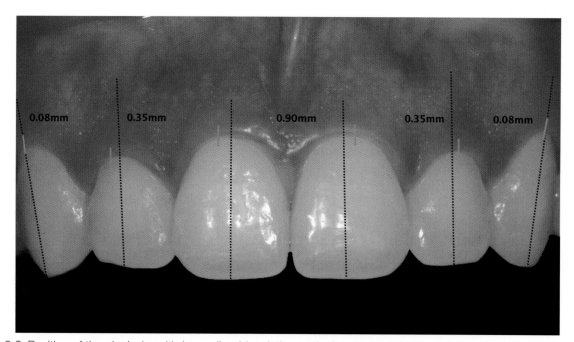

0.08mm   0.35mm   0.90mm   0.35mm   0.08mm

Figure 9.2 Position of the gingival zenith (green lines) in relation to the long axis of the teeth (black dashed lines).

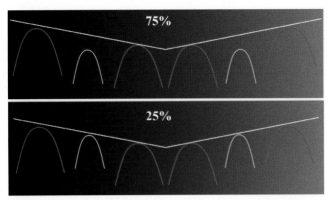

Figure 9.3 Marginal soft tissue level. The gingival zenith of the lateral incisor is either located coronally or level with the zenith line of the adjacent central incisor and canine.

MARGINAL SOFT TISSUE LEVEL

Coronal Displacement of the Lateral Incisor Zenith

The majority of the population (70%) present with the gingival margin of the lateral incisor positioned coronally to the zeniths of the ipsi-lateral canines and central incisors, while in 30% of the population the gingival margin of the lateral incisors is positioned at the same level of the zeniths of the ipsi-lateral canines and central incisors (Mattos & Santana 2008) (Fig. 9.3). In no instance is the lateral incisor positioned apically to the neighboring teeth. The coronal displacement of the zenith of the lateral incisors amounts to a mean of 0.75 ± 0.60 mm (minimum 0.14 mm, maximum 2.6 mm) (Fig. 9.4).

Interdental Papilla

The physiologic gingival architecture is characterized by a "parabolic shape flowing smoothly from the conical interdental area, which is positioned coronally to the buccal and lingual (or palatal) plates of bone, following the shape of the cementoenamel junction" (Prichard 1961). Thus, a thin, scalloped, knife-edged gingival contour with pyramid-shaped

papillae that fill the interproximal space (Bensimon 1999) is established.

The interdental papilla (IP) is the gingival tissue, which occupies the embrasure space beneath the contact area of two adjacent teeth (Fig. 9.5). It is assumed that, in anterior segments of the dentition, the IP presents with conical or pyramidal forms depending on the width of the interdental space. The papillary width (PW) is measured as the horizontal distance between the gingival zeniths located immediately mesially and distally (Fig. 9.5). The papillary height (PH) is measured as the vertical distance from the bisector point of PH to the tip of the papilla (Fig. 9.5).

The lateral borders and tips of the dental papilla are formed by marginal gingiva, and the intervening portion consists of attached gingiva. Thus, histologically, the IP is composed of dense connective tissue covered by oral epithelium. The shape of the IP is determined by the contact relationships between the teeth, the width of the approximal tooth surfaces and the course of the cemento-enamel junction (CEJ) (Lindhe et al. 2008). Various factors may influence the presence or absence of the IP. These include crestal alveolar bone height, the dimensions of the interproximal space, soft tissue appearance, buccal plate thickness, and contact area (Deepalakshmi et al. 2007).

A significant relationship between either the interdental contact point or the interdental distance and the presence, size, and shape of the interdental papilla has been reported (Tal 1984; Heins & Wieder 1986; Tarnow et al. 1992; Cho et al. 2006; Ferreira-Lopes et al. 2008; Chu et al. 2009; Stappert et al. 2010; Nozawa et al. 2011) and is considered to be an important factor in esthetic dentistry (Nozawa et al. 2011) since, theoretically, it defines the height of the interdental papilla (Stappert et al. 2010). Tarnow et al. (1992) demonstrated that the interdental papilla was present almost 100% of the time when the distance from the contact point to the crest of the bone was 5 mm or less. Ferreira-Lopes et al. (2008) demonstrated that the distance between the base of the contact point and

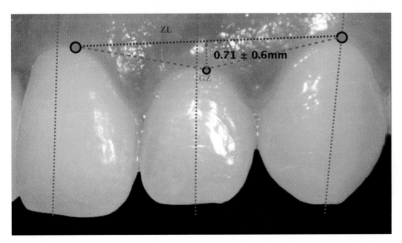

Figure 9.4 The gingival zenith (GZ) of the lateral incisor is located coronally to the zenith line (ZL) connecting the gingival zenith of the adjacent central incisor and canine.

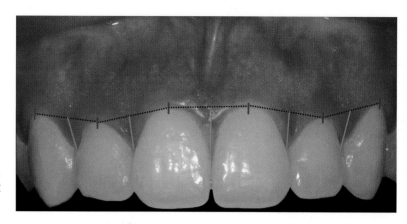

Figure 9.5 Papilla dimension measurement. Papillary width (black dotted line), papillary height (green lines), and gingival zenith (blue lines).

the most coronal portion of the bone crest was correlated with the degree of vertical loss on the interdental papilla in humans (Fig. 9.6). Based on these findings, the relationship between the contact point and bone crest has been widely used (1) to evaluate the interproximal area as a prognostic factor for interdental papilla formation following treatment (Bichacho 1998; Prato et al. 2004; Zetu & Wang 2005; Cho et al. 2006; Chu et al. 2009; Nozawa et al. 2011), (2) to classify the presence or absence of interproximal papilla (Nordland & Tarnow 1998; Cardaropoli et al. 2004), and (3) to act as a pre-surgical evaluation in periodontal plastic reconstructive surgeries (Deepalakshmi et al. 2007).

Clinical studies have proposed ideal relationships between the distance between bone crest and contact point, and the length of the clinical crown as measured from the incisal edge (LaVacca et al. 2005; Chu et al. 2009), thus establishing a relationship between an internal landmark (distance from bone crest to contact point) and an external measurement of the length of the clinical crown. Clinical perceptional research has proposed that an ideal aesthetic position of the interdental papilla should be between 50% and 70% of the length of the clinical crown as measured from the incisal edge (La Vacca

et al. 2005; Chu et al. 2009), and that the crown length, measured from the bone crest to the incisal edge, is 3–5 mm greater (average 4 mm) than the most coronal aspect of the interdental papilla (Chu et al. 2009). A closer-to-ideal spatial relationship between teeth and their respective papillae can be established to achieve optimized esthetics by mathematically quantifying the papilla length from the gingival zenith (Chu et al. 2009). Mean papilla proportions were approximately 42.5% of the clinical crown length as measured from the level of the gingival zenith (Chu et al. 2009). The measured mesial and distal papilla proportions on the central incisor, lateral incisor, and canine were 41% and 42%, 41% and 41%, and 43% and 45%, respectively.

Some studies have reported that the interproximal distance is an important determinant of the IP height (Chang et al. 1999; Touati 1995; Cho et al. 2006), thus affecting the appearance of the hard and soft tissues in the embrasure space. However, data from the maxillary anterior region is scarce. Cho et al. (2006) reported that the ideal horizontal dimension for the existence of papillae was 1.5–2.5 mm between adjacent roots. According to Cardaropoli et al. (2004), the formation of pathologic diastema, without the presence of a normal contact point, creates the presupposing situation for an apical shift of the interproximal papilla. In the presence of diastema, when the proximal contours of adjacent teeth are too far from each other, the interdental papilla may be visibly absent because a round or flat papillary tip is observed (Fig. 9.7) instead of a triangular shape (Bichacho 1998). The absence or loss of interdental papillae, resulting in so-called "black triangles" (Figs. 9.6 and 9.7), may create aesthetic impairments, phonetic problems, and food impaction (Tarnow et al. 1992; Kokich 1996), which result in important clinical problems.

PERIODONTAL PHENOTYPE: TOOTH CROWN/GINGIVA RELATIONSHIPS

The specific morphologies and relationships of the interdental soft tissues, bone, and tooth surfaces have been described. In this regard, Hirschfeld reported in 1923 that a thin alveolar bone contour is probably covered with a thin gingival form.

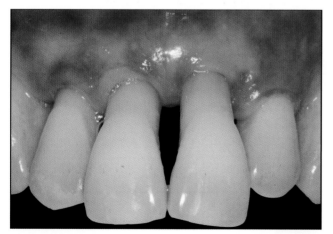

Figure 9.6 Interdental soft tissue recession leading to the loss of the interdental papillae.

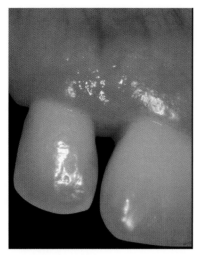

Figure 9.7 Flat papillary tip observed is area with a diastema.

Ochsenbein & Ross (1969) identified two distinct normal gingival architectures, scalloped and flat, which influence the papillary length. The marginal gingival contour is also affected by the degree of concavity and convexity of the tooth surface. The higher the convexity of the root surface, the more markedly scalloped is the gingival margin, therefore specific relationships between tooth morphology and gingival architecture have been proposed. Weisgold (1977) recognized that the gingival tissues are thicker in the flat as compared with the scalloped gingival form (Fig. 9.8A,B). This author also noted that specific

tooth forms exist for each of the aforementioned gingival forms. The scalloped gingival type was associated with longer papillae and short, incisally located interproximal contact areas, while the flat gingival type had short papillae and long interproximal contact areas. It was observed that gingival tissues in a scalloped periodontium are generally thinner than in a flat periodontium (Weisgold 1977).

These concepts have been widely employed in many aspects of clinical periodontology. The gingival type apparently influences the amount of attached gingiva (Weisgold 1977), tissue response to injury (Weisgold 1977; Olsson & Lindhe 1991), rebound healing following crown lengthening surgery (Pontoriero & Carnevale 2001), presence or absence of interproximal papillae (Zetu & Wang 2005), risk of papillary recession following tooth extraction (Kois 2001), root coverage following periodontal plastic surgery (Saletta et al. 2001; Berlucchi et al. 2005), and the dimension of the peri-implant mucosa following second-stage surgery (Kan et al. 2003). Tissue biotypes are therefore considered to be related to the outcomes of periodontal therapy, conventional prosthodontics, implant therapy, and root coverage procedures (Fu et al. 2010; Cook et al. 2011).

Gingival areas clinically classified as thin, based on the transparency of the gingival tissues (Fig. 9.9), exhibited significantly thinner gingival tissues (de Rouck et al. 2009; Kan et al. 2010; Fu et al. 2010; Cook et al. 2011). Earlier studies (Aimetti et al. 2008; Kan et al. 2010) quantified gingival tissue by classifying thin as ≤1.0 mm and thick as >1.0 mm. Other studies

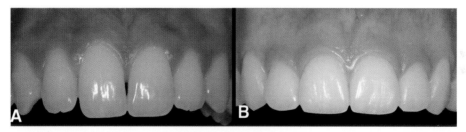

Figure 9.8 Periodontal phenotypes: (A) thin and scalloped; (B) thick and flat (note the classical pale coral color).

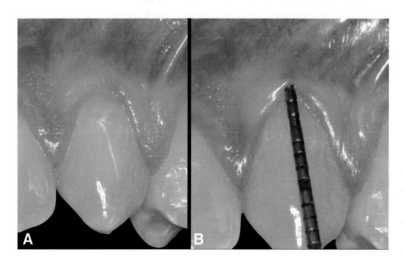

Figure 9.9 A thin gingival phenotype (A) may be clinically determined by the transparence of the gingival tissues (B). Note that the periodontal probe tip can be seen through the gingival transparence (B).

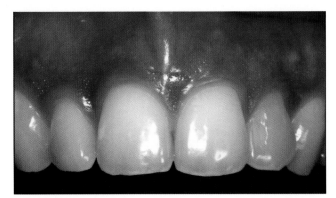

Figure 9.10 In patients with physiologic melanin pigmentation, the gingival tissues present with brownish color.

employing ultrasonic technology revealed that the mean gingival tissue ranged from 0.63 ± 0.11 mm to 1.79 ± 0.31 mm (Eger et al. 1996; Muller et al. 2007). In surgical root coverage procedures, a critical threshold of >1.1 mm of gingival tissue was reported for predictable complete root coverage (Hwang & Wang 2006) and gingival tissue >1.44 mm appears to indicate stability of tissue after surgery (Zuhr et al. 2014). Thus, increasing the gingival tissue to values thicker than 1.5 mm may mitigate the negative effects of a thin biotype.

GINGIVAL COLOR

The color of the gingival tissues may vary between pale coral (Fig. 9.8B) and pink to brown (in patients with higher degrees of physiological melanin pigmentation) (Fig. 9.10), and is influenced by the degree of queratinization, local vasculature, pigmentation, and epithelial thickness in the area (Stern 1986). Areas with a well-developed and thick keratinized epithelium layer, such as in the gingiva (Fig. 9.11), tend to disguise the underlying vasculature and thus present a paler color when compared with the darker red colored alveolar mucosa (Figs. 9.11–9.13), which present a thinner, less keratinized epithelium and loose connective tissue (Fig. 9.11). Similarly, the palatal mucosa generally presents with thicker, more queratinized, epithelium and denser connective tissue, therefore, when transplanted to areas of alveolar mucosa or thin, delicate, gingival tissues the grafted area may exhibit a whitish color. These aspects should be taken in consideration when planning for soft tissue grafting in the aesthetic areas, especially if the tissue to be grafted contains the epithelial layer of the donor area, such as performed in the free gingival graft procedure.

GINGIVAL SUPERFICIAL TEXTURE AND CONSISTENCY

The gingival tissues present a firm consistency. The marginal gingiva has a smooth surface and can be easily retracted away from the tooth, while the attached gingiva presents with delicate superficial depressions, called "stippling" (Fig. 9.12), and is firmly attached to the underlying bone and cementum. The gingival stippling is present in 40% of individuals (Ainamo & Löe 1966), but even if present may not be uniformly

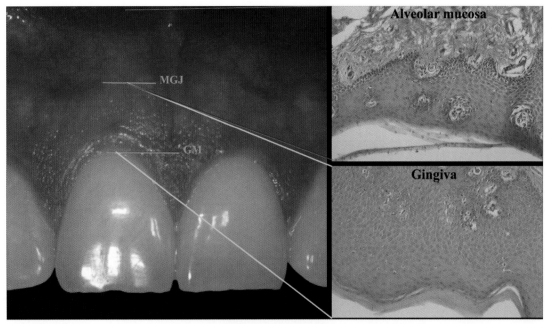

Figure 9.11 Clinical and histologic comparison between the gingiva and the alveolar mucosa. The gingiva is limited coronally by the gingival margin (GM) and apically by the muco-gingival junction (MGJ), which continues apically as the darker reddish, smooth, highly elastic alveolar mucosa.

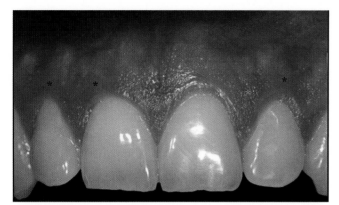

Figure 9.12 The marginal gingiva and areas of the attached gingiva (black stars) have a smooth surface, while the other areas (green stars) of the attached gingiva present with superficial depressions (stippling), which are not seen in every individual and are not uniformly distributed within the same individual.

distributed (Fig. 9.12). The smooth alveolar (lining) mucosa is loosely bound to the underlying bone and highly elastic, making it mobile in relation to the underlying tissues (Figs. 9.11 and 9.13).

GINGIVAL DIMENSIONS

The free gingiva demonstrates a width of 0.5–1.0 mm determined by the existence of the gingival sulcus, which measures between 0 and 3 mm clinically with the use of a probe (Goldman 1950), or between 0.69 mm (Gargiullo et al. 1961) and 1.21 mm (Stanley 1955) histologically. The width of the attached gingiva varies in different regions of the mouth between 1 and 9 mm (Ainamo & Löe 1966). It is widest in the anterior segments and narrower in the posterior areas. In the anterior maxillary sextant the width of the gingiva varies between 2.0 and 10.0 mm, with a mean width of 5.5 ± 1.6 mm and the widest band located in the lateral incisor area (Ainamo & Löe 1966; Miranda 2005). In the mandible, the width of keratinized tissue in lingual aspect varies from 1 to 8 mm (Voight et al. 1978). The wider (mean 4.7 mm) zone of attached gingiva is located in the molar areas and the narrowest (mean 1.9 mm) in the incisors and canines (Voight et al. 1978).

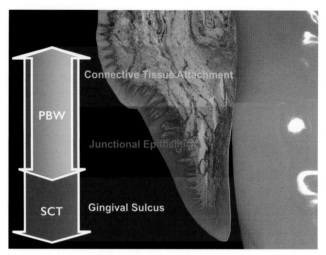

Figure 9.14 Periodontal biologic width (PBW) and supracrestal gingival tissues (SCT). The PBW is the distance between the base of the gingival sulcus and the top of the alveolar bone crest and thus is composed of the junctional epithelium and the connective tissue attachment. The supracrestal gingival tissues (SCT) extend from the bone crest to the gingival margin and correspond to the length of the gingival sulcus added to the PBW.

PERIODONTAL BIOLOGIC WIDTH

Sicher (1959) described a type of gingival attachment, the dento-gingival junction, as a functional unit composed of gingival connective tissue attachment and epithelial adhesion. Cohen (1959), based on the histometric measurements performed by Gargiulo et al. (1961), named the distance between the most coronal aspect of the junctional epithelium and the alveolar bone crest (BC) as the biologic width. Currently, the distance between the base of the gingival sulcus and the top of the alveolar bone crest is called the periodontal biologic width (PBW) and is composed of two zones surrounding the tooth, the junctional epithelium and the connective tissue attachment (Fig. 9.14), which acts as a protective barrier against the invasion of bacteria and its by-products.

The dimensions of the PBW components have been measured histometrically in humans (Stanley 1955; Gargiulo et al. 1961; Vacek et al. 1994). The dimensions of the junctional epithelium

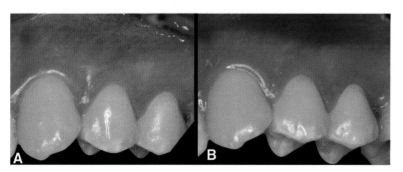

Figure 9.13 With the use of histochemical methods, the alveolar mucosa is stained brown, allowing clear definition of the muco-gingival junction and, thus, separation of the alveolar mucosa and gingiva.

varied between 0.38 and 2.48 mm (Vacek et al. 1994), while the connective tissue attachment varied between 0.35 and 1.34 mm (Vacek et al. 1994). Thus, the mean dimensions of the PBW varied, in different studies, between 1.50 mm (Stanley 1955), 1.75 ± 0.56 mm (Vacek et al. 1994), and 2.04 mm (Gargiulo et al. 1961). Traditionally, the measurements reported by Gargiulo et al. (1961) are used for the PBW.

Supra-Crestal Soft Tissues

The soft tissues surrounding the teeth that extend from the BC to the gingival margin (GM) are named supra-crestal tissues (SCT) and correspond to the the total dimension composed of the PBW and the gingival sulcus (Santana et al. 2013) (Fig. 9.14). Although divergent definitions are found in the literature (Nevins & Skurrow 1984), the gingival sulcus is *not* a component of the PBW (Fig. 9.14). Despite its significant relevance, the PBW is a histologic bio-morphometric concept, and thus impossible to measure by conventional clinical means. In contrast, the SCT includes the totality of the soft tissues located coronally to the BC, allowing clinical measurements with the use of trans-sulcular probing under anaesthesia (Miranda 2005). The measurement of the SCT is therefore an important, easily performed, and reproducible clinical resource for clinical diagnosis, and should not be confused with the dimensions of the PBW.

REFERENCES

Aimetti, M., Massei, G., Morra, M., Cardesi, E., & Romano, F. (2008) Correlation between gingival phenotype and Schneiderian membrane thickness. *International Journal of Oral Maxillofacial Implants* 23, 1128–1132.

Ainamo, J., & Löe, H. (1966) Anatomical characteristics of gingiva. A clinical and microscopic study of the free and attached gingiva. *Journal of Periodontology* 37, 5–13.

Allen, A.P. (1988) Use of mucogingival surgical procedures to enhance esthetics. *Dental Clinic of North America* 32, 307–330.

Bensimon, G.C. (1999) Surgical crown-lengthening procedure to enhance esthetics. *The International Journal of Periodontics and Restorative Dentistry* 19(4), 332–341.

Berlucchi, I., Francetti, L., del Fabbro, M., Basso, M., & Weinstein, R.L. (2005) The influence of anatomical features on the outcome of gingival recessions treated with coronally advanced flap and enamel matrix derivative: a 1-year prospective study. *Journal of Periodontology* 76, 899–907.

Bichacho, N. (1998) Papilla regeneration by noninvasive prosthodontic treatment: Segmental proximal restorations. *Practical Periodontics and Aesthetic Dentistry* 10, 75, 77–78.

Borguetti, A., & Monnet-Corti, V. (2002) *Periodontal Plastic Surgery* [Portuguese]. Artmed Ed, Porto Alegre, pp. 105–107.

Cardaropoli, D., Re, S., & Corrente, G. (2004) The Papilla Presence Index (PPI): a new system to assess interproximal papillary levels. *The International Journal of Periodontics and Restorative Dentistry* 24, 488–492.

Chang, M., Wennström, J.L., Ödman, P., & Andersson, B. (1999) Implant supported single-tooth replacements compared to contralateral natural teeth. Crown and soft tissue dimensions. *Clinical Oral Implants Research* 10, 185–194.

Cho, H.S., Jang, H.S., Kim, D.K., Park, J.C., Kim, H.J., Choi, S.H., Kim, C.K., & Kim, B.O. (2006) The effect of interproximal distance between roots on the existence of interdental papillae according to the distance from the contact point to the alveolar crest. *Journal of Periodontology* Oct., 1651–1657.

Chu, S.J., Tarnow, D.P., Tan, J.H., & Stappert, C.F. (2009) Papilla proportions in the maxillary anterior dentition. *The International Journal of Periodontics and Restorative Dentistry* 29, 385–393.

Cohen, B. (1959) Morphological factors in the pathogenesis of periodontal disease. *British Dentistry Journal* 107, 31–39.

Cook, D.R., Mealey, B.L., Verrett, R.G., Mills, M.P., Noujeim, M.E., Lasho, D.J., & Cronin Jr, R.J. (2011) Relationship between clinical periodontal biotype and labial plate thickness: an in vivo study. *The International Journal of Periodontics and Restorative Dentistry* 31, 345–354.

Deepalaksmi, D., Ahathya, R.S., Raja, S., & Kumar, A. (2007) Surgical reconstruction of lost interdental papilla: a case report. *Quintessence International* 4(3), 229–334.

de Rouck, T., Eghbali, R., Collys, K., de Bruyn, H., & Cosyn, J. (2009) The gingival biotype revisited: transparency of the periodontal probe through the gingival margin as a method to discriminate thin from thick gingiva. *Journal of Clinical Periodontology* 36, 428–433.

Eger, T., Muller, H.P., & Heinecke, A. (1996) Ultrasonic determination of gingival thickness. Subject variation and influence of tooth type and clinical features. *Journal of Clinical Periodontology* 23, 839–845.

Ferreira-Lopes, M.W., Gusmão, E.S., Alves, R.V., Rosing, C.K., & Cimões, R. (2008) Effect of the distance from the contact point to the crestal bone on the degree of vertical loss of interdental papillae. *Perio* 5(2), 117–120.

Fu, J.H., Yeh, C.Y., Chan, H.L., Tatarakis, N., Leong, D.J., & Wang, H.L. (2010) Tissue biotype and its relation to the underlying bone morphology. *Journal of Periodontology* 81, 569–574.

Gargiulo, A.W., Wentz, F.M., & Orban, B. (1961) Dimensions and relations of the dentogingival junctions in humans. *Journal of Periodontology* 32(3), 261–267.

Goldman, H.M. (1950) The development of physiologic gingival contours by gingivoplasty. *Oral Surgery, Oral Medicine, Oral Pathology* 3, 879–888.

Grant, D.A., Stern, I.B., & Listgarten, M.A. (1988) *Periodontics. In the Tradition of Gottlieb and Orban*, 6th edn. C.V. Mosby Co., St Louis, pp. 4–10.

Heins, P.J., & Wieder, S.M. (1986) A histologic study of the width and nature of inter-radicular spaces in human adult pre-molars and molars. *Journal of Dental Research* February, 948–951.

Hirschfeld, I. (1923) A study of skulls in the American Museum of Natural History in relation to periodontal disease. *Journal of Dental Research* 5, 241–265.

Hwang, D., & Wang, H.L. (2006) Flap thickness as a predictor of root coverage: a systematic review. *Journal of Periodontology* 77, 1625–1634.

Kan, J.Y., Rungcharasseeng, K., Umezu, K., & Kois, J.C. (2003) Dimensions of peri-implant mucosa: an evaluation of maxillary anterior single implants in humans. *Journal of Periodontology* 74, 557–562.

Kan, J.Y., Morimoto, T., Rungcharassaeng, K., Roe, P., & Smith, D.H. (2010) Gingival biotype assessment in the esthetic zone: visual versus direct measurement. *The International Journal of Periodontics and Restorative Dentistry* 30(3), 237–243.

Kay, H.B. (1982) Esthetic considerations in the definitive periodontal prosthetic management of the maxillary anterior segment. *The International Journal of Periodontics and Restorative Dentistry* 2(3), 45–59.

Kois, J.C. (2001) Predictable single tooth peri-implant esthetics: Five diagnostic keys. *Compendium of Continuing Education in Dentistry* 22, 199–206; quiz 208.

Kokich, V.G. (1996) Esthetics: The orthodontic-periodontic restorative connection. *Seminars in Orthodontics* 2, 21–30.

LaVacca, M.I., Tarnow, D.P., & Cisneros, G.J. (2005) Interdental papilla length and the perception of aesthetics. *Practical Procedures and Aesthetic Dentistry* 17, 405–412.

Lindhe, J., Lang, N.P., & Karring, K. (2008) *Periodontology and Implant Dentistry*, 5th edn. Blackwell Munksgaard, Oxford, p. 6.

Löe, H., Listgarten, M.A., & Terranova, V.P. (1990) The gingiva: structure and function, in *Contemporary Periodontics* (eds R.J. Genco, H.M. Goldman, and D.W. Cohen). St Louis, C.V. Mosby Co., pp. 3–32.

Magne, P., & Belser, U. (2002) *Bonded porcelain restorations in the anterior dentition: a biomimetic approach*. Quintessence Publishing Co, Inc., Chicago, pp. 57–98.

Mattos, C.M., & Santana, R.B. (2008) A quantitative evaluation of the spatial displacement of the gingival zenith in the maxillary anterior dentition. *Journal of Periodontology* 79(10), 1880–1885.

Melcher, A.H., & Bowen, W.H. (1969) *Biology of the Periodontium*. Academic Press, London, p. 107.

Miranda, J.L.C. (2005) Evaluation of the supracrestal tissues in clinically-healthy periodontium in young adults. Thesis (Master of Science in Dentistry), Dental School – Federal Fluminense University, 63pp.

Morr, T. (2004) Understanding the esthetic evaluation for success. *Journal of the California Dental Association* 32(2), 153–160.

Muller, H.P., Barrieshi-Nusair, K.M., & Kononen, E. (2007) Repeatability of ultrasonic determination of gingival thickness. *Clinical Oral Investigations* 11, 439–442.

Nevins, M., & Skurow, H.M. (1984) The intracrevicular restorative margin, the biologic width, and the maintenance of the gingival margin. *The International Journal of Periodontics and Restorative Dentistry* 4, 30–49.

Nordland, W.P., & Tarnow, D.P. (1998) A classification system for loss of papillary height. *Journal of Periodontology* 69, 1124–1126.

Nozawa, T., Yamaguchi, S., Ookame, Y., Shimada, K., Tanaka, K., & Ito, K. (2011) The distances between the facial and palatal papillae in the maxillary anterior dentition. *European Journal of Esthetic Dentistry* 6(1), 88–93.

Ochsenbein, C., & Ross, S. (1969) A reevaluation of osseous surgery. *Dental Clinics of North America* 13, 87–102.

Olsson, M., & Lindhe, J. (1991) Periodontal characteristics in individuals with varying form of the upper central incisors. *Journal of Clinical Periodontology* 18, 78–82.

Pontoriero, R., & Carnevale, G. (2001) Surgical crown lengthening: a 12-month clinical wound healing study. *Journal of Periodontology* 72, 841–848.

Prato, G.P., Rotundo, R., Cortellini, P., Tinti, C., & Azzi, R. (2004) Interdental papilla management: A review and classification of the therapeutic approaches. *International Journal of Periodontics and Restorative Dentistry* 24, 246–255.

Prichard, J. (1961) Gingivoplasty, gingivectomy and osseous surgery. *Journal of Periodontology* 32, 275–282.

Rufenacht, C. (1990) *Fundamentals of Esthetics*. Quintessence Publishing Co., Inc., Chicago, pp. 124–127.

Saletta, D., Pini Prato, G., Pagliaro, U., Baldi, C., Mauri, M., & Nieri, M. (2001) Coronally advanced flap procedure: is the interdental papilla a prognostic factor for root coverage? *Journal of Periodontology* 72, 760–766.

Santana, R.B., Santana, C.M.M., & Miranda, J.L.C. (2013) *Clinical Excellence in Oral Implantology*, Vol. 1. Quintessence Publishing Co., Inc., São Paulo, p. 352.

Schroeder, H.E. (1986) *The Periodontium*. Springer-Verlag, Berlin, pp. 238–247.

Schroeder, H.E. (1991) *Oral Structural Biology*. Thieme Medical Publishers, Inc., New York, pp. 230–232.

Sicher, H. (1959) Changing concepts of the supporting dental structures. *Oral Surgery Oral Medicine Oral Pathology* 12(1), 31–35.

Silvestri, L. (2002) Cosmetic dentistry: Aesthetics in the anterior zone: What are the considerations prior to treatment? *Oral Health and Dental Practice Management* [serial online] April. Accessed 24 November 2007.

Smallwood, T.W. (2003) *Contemporary Esthetics Platinum Paradigm*. Visual Smile Creations, Phoenix, pp. 2–20.

Stanley, H.S. (1955) The cyclic phenomenon of periodontitis. *Oral Surgery* 8(5), 598–610.

Stappert, C.F., Tarnow, D.P., Tan, J.H., & Chu, S.J. (2010) Proximal contact areas of the maxillary anterior dentition. *International Journal of Periodontics and Restorative Dentistry* 30, 471–477.

Stein, R.S. (1977) The ceramo-metal restoration. Presented before the Alpha Omega Sunshine Seminar, Miami 1977, *apud* Kay, H.B. Esthetic considerations in the definitive periodontal prosthetic management of the maxillary anterior segment. *International Journal of Periodontics and Restorative Dentistry* 1982 2(3), 45–59.

Stern, I.B. (1986) Oral mucous membrane. In *Orbans's Oral Histology and Embryology*, 10th edn (ed S.N. Bhaskar). Mosby Co., St Louis.

Tal, H. (1984) Relationship between the interproximal distance of roots and the prevalence of bony pockets. *Journal of Periodontology* 55, 604–607.

Tarnow, D.P., Magner, A.W., & Fletcher, P. (1992) The effect of the distance from the contact point to the crest of bone on the presence or absence of the interproximal dental papilla. *Journal of Periodontology* 63, 995–996.

Touati, B. (1995) Improving aesthetics of implant-supported restorations. *Practical Procedings in Aesthetic Dentistry* 7, 81–93.

Vacek, J.S., Gher, M.E., Assad, D.A., Richardson, A.C., & Giambarresi, L.I. (1994) The dimensions of the human dentogingival junction. *Practical Procedures in Aesthetic Dentistry* 14(2), 154–165.

Voight, J.P., Goran, M.L., & Fleisher, R.M. (1978) The width of lingual mandibular attached gingiva. *Journal of Periodontology* 49(2), 77–80.

Weisgold, A.S. (1977) Contours of the full crown restoration. *Alpha Omegan* 70, 77–89.

Zetu, L., & Wang, H.L. (2005) Management of inter-dental/inter-implant papilla. *Journal of Clinical Periodontology* 32, 831–839.

Zuhr, O., Baumer, D., & Hurzeler, M. (2014) The addition of soft tissue replacement grafts in plastic periodontal and implant surgery: critical elements in design and execution. *Journal of Clinical Periodontology* 41(Suppl. 15), S123–S142.

Chapter 10 Enamel Matrix Derivative: Emdogain

Ronaldo B. Santana and Serge Dibart

INTRODUCTION

Emdogain

Enamel matrix derivative (EMD) is prepared from an acidic extract of homogenized extracellular matrix from tooth buds of swine, and contains predominantly the protein amelogenin as well as other enamel matrix proteins and growth factors such as transforming growth factor beta (Kawase et al. 2001; Venezia et al. 2004). Emdogain consists of the sterilized and lyophilized amelogenin fraction of porcine enamel matrix, dissolved in propylene glycol alginate (PGA) (Venezia et al. 2004). After application, EMD precipitates on the root surface forming aggregated microspheres (Gestrelius et al. 1997a), and active enamel proteins are continuously released for several weeks thereafter (Sculean et al. 2002).

Biological Actions

Culturing studies in vitro have demonstrated that EMD affects cellular attachment, proliferation, biosynthesis, and differentiation (Kalpidis & Ruben 2002). EMD acts selectively on periodontal ligament fibroblasts and stimulates attachment, proliferation, extracellular matrix synthesis, autocrine growth factor expression, and cellular differentiation (Gestrelius et al. 1997b; van der Paw et al. 2000; Haase & Barthold 2001; Lyngstadaas et al. 2001; Hoang et al. 2002). In addition, EMD may also regulate the activity of osteoblastic and cementoblastic cells (Schwartz et al. 2000; Tokiyasu et al. 2000; Jiang et al. 2001; Ohyama et al. 2002), while exhibiting a cytostatic effect on epithelial cells in vitro (Gestrelius et al. 1997b; Kawase et al. 2001). Taken together, these effects support the notion that EMD selectively stimulates the cells responsible for bone, cementum, and periodontal ligament regeneration, as extensively documented histologically in animals and humans (Castellanos et al. 2006).

CLINICAL ADVANTAGES

Recession defects treated with Emdogain® (Straumann, Switzerland), in conjunction with the coronally advanced flap (CAF) procedure, exhibited significantly enhanced mean root coverage and keratinized tissue width, smaller areas of exposed root surfaces, and complete root coverage obtained more frequently (McGuire et al. 2012; Cueva et al. 2004; Spahr et al. 2005; Castellanos et al. 2006; Moses et al. 2006). Longitudinal studies have demonstrated that CAF plus Emdogain presented equivalent results to CAF plus connective tissue graft in the treatment of single recession defects up to 10 years after treatment (McGuire et al. 2012). Additionally, recession areas treated with Emdogain may heal with true periodontal regeneration via the formation of new cementum, periodontal ligament, and alveolar bone (McGuire & Cochran 2003; Castellanos et al. 2006). Thus, addition of Emdogain to the surgical coverage of root recession defects may present a less invasive treatment approach by eliminating the need for graft procurement and, therefore, limiting patient morbidity.

INDICATIONS

- Single or multiple adjacent recessions that have adequate donor tissue apically (root coverage)

- Single or multiple adjacent recessions without adequate donor tissue apically (root coverage) when used in conjunction with a connective tissue graft

PREREQUISITES

- Miller class I gingival recession: single or multiple

- Thick periodontal biotype

- Preferably deep vestibule

ARMAMENTARIUM

The basic surgical kit for periodontal plastic surgery includes:

- Gracey (Hu-Friedy, Chicago, IL) curette #1/2

- Scalpel handle mounted with surgical blade no. 15C

- Wide-field surgical loupes (4.5X)

- PrefGel (Straumann, Switzerland)

Practical Periodontal Plastic Surgery, Second Edition. Edited by Serge Dibart.
© 2017 John Wiley & Sons, Inc. Published 2017 by John Wiley & Sons, Inc.

Titanium instruments for microsurgery:

- Two straight forceps
- One straight strong forceps
- One curved needle holder with lock
- One straight scissors
- P-1 needle with a 7-0 coated vicryl suture

TECHNICAL PROCEDURES

Flap Design

The flap is produced by performing two vertical releasing incisions at the mesial and distal aspects of the recession to be treated, in such a way that the proximal papillae are not included as part of the flap (Allen & Miller 1989). Papillae are never bisected. Beveled divergent vertical incisions are performed in the attached gingiva, initiating at the CEJ level on the mesial and distal line angles of the tooth, avoiding the formation of butt joints between the flap and adjacent tissues, and are continued several millimeters apically into the alveolar mucosa.

The vertical incisions are joined by an intrasulcular incision. In the interproximal area, the papillae are split in a mesio-distal dimension, resulting in a flat surface of connective tissue for contact between the flap tissues and the retained portion of the papillae after repositioning and suturing of the flap. A combined mucoperiosteal–mucosal trapezoidal flap is elevated such that the first 3–4 mm coronal aspect of the alveolar bone is exposed, while the remaining buccal bone is still covered by the periosteum and gingival connective tissue. A complementary horizontal incision is performed on the apical aspect of the flap, by means of partial-thickness dissection, releasing the flap from the attached periosteum and muscle fibers. This allows the elongation and free coronal positioning of the flap. Roots are prepared as described below. The flap is then positioned at least 1 mm coronal to the CEJ and kept in place by individual 5.0 monofilament sutures.

Envelope Technique

The procedure is designed as a split–full-split thickness envelope flap (Zucchelli & de Sanctis 2000). A horizontal incision consisting of oblique submarginal incisions is performed in the interdental areas, at both the mesial and distal aspects of the recession to be treated. It is then joined in an intrasulcular incision at the recession defects. The papillary portion located coronally to the oblique interdental incisions is de-epithelized, while the papillary portion located apically to the oblique incision is split in a mesio-distal dimension, resulting in a flat surface of connective tissue for contact between the flap tissues and the retained portion of the papillae after repositioning and suturing of the flap. A combined mucoperiosteal–mucosal envelope

flap is elevated such that the first 3–4 mm coronal aspect of the alveolar bone is exposed, while the remaining buccal bone is still covered by the periosteum and gingival connective tissue. A complementary horizontal incision is performed on the apical aspect of the flap by means of partial-thickness dissection, releasing the flap from the attached periosteum and muscle fibers. This allows elongation and free coronal positioning of the flap. Roots are prepared as described below. The flap is then positioned at least 1 mm coronal to the CEJ and kept in place by individual 5.0 monofilament sutures.

Root Preparation

After flap elevation and periosteal release, thorough root planning is performed with hand and ultrasonic instruments in all treated sites. A fine-grain finishing bur (Perio-Set, Intensiv S.A, Grancia, Switzerland) is used to remove sharp edges and grooves, and for root polishing. After instrumentation, the root surfaces are washed with saline solution to remove any remaining detached fragments from the defect and surgical field. The root surfaces are then conditioned with a 24% EDTA gel (PrefGel®, Straumann, Switzerland) for 2 min and thoroughly rinsed with sterile saline. This initial procedure aims to enhance the biocompatibility of the instrumented root surfaces by successfully removing the radicular smear layer and exposing the collagenous matrix of the root surface without inducing necrosis of the periodontal ligament. The root surfaces are then conditioned with Emdogain®. Extreme care is taken to avoid contamination of the root surfaces with blood after the EDTA root conditioning and during the first 2 or 3 min after the application of Emdogain® in order to optimize the deposition and effects of the product. After this period, blood contamination may be less critical. The gel should be kept in place and not be aspirated or washed out of the root surfaces. Additional procedures that are to be performed, such as connective tissue graft placement and/or suturing, are then completed.

POST-SURGICAL CARE

The surgical dressing (CoePak, IL, USA) is changed after 7 days and removed after 14 days. Patients are put on systemic analgesics for 4 days and instructed to continue their regular home hygiene care, except in the operated area, in which toothbrushing is discontinued for the first 30 days after surgery and plaque control is maintained by gentle topical applications of chlorhexidine gluconate (0.2%) on saturated cotton swabs twice a day. Gentle tooth-brushing with an extra-soft-bristle toothbrush is then initiated. Analgesics are prescribed on an individual basis. The sutures are removed 2 weeks after the surgery.

Maintenance Schedule

Following surgery, patients are seen weekly during the first 3 months and bi-weekly for the next 3 months. Maintenance visits consist of reinforcement of oral hygiene procedures and professional supra-gingival coronal polishing. Additional oral chemical plaque control is performed once every 3 months by means of mouth rinses with a solution of chlorhexidine gluconate 0.12% BID for 1 week.

Wound Healing

Healing in areas of gingival recession treated by coronally advanced flap and Emdogain heal by regeneration of the periodontal attachment apparatus, including alveolar bone, new cementum, and periodontal ligament (McGuire & Cochran 2003; Castellanos et al. 2006). The area should not be probed or scaled for 6 months, as these procedures may destroy the regenerating attachment apparatus (Hatekayama et al. 2005). Coverage of the exposed root surfaces with this technique has varied from 73.2% to 95.1% (McGuire & Nunn 2003; Cueva et al. 2004; Spahr et al. 2005; Castellanos et al. 2006; Moses et al. 2006; McGuire et al. 2012).

POSSIBLE LIMITATIONS AND COMPLICATIONS

The most common limitation is a slight residual recession at the treated site, although this is observed significantly less frequently than in equivalent procedures without the use of Emdogain® (Cuevas et al. 2004; Spahr et al. 2005; Moses et al. 2006).

Possible complications include necrosis or loosening of the flap. This happens if the flap is too thin, in a partial thickness flap, or because of faulty technique or inadequate anatomy. The flap will loosen if the dissection was insufficient and the flap was sutured with tension. It should be emphasized, however, that these complications are relatively rare.

REFERENCES

Allen, E.P., & Miller, P.D. Jr. (1989) Coronal positioning of existing gingiva: short term results in the treatment of shallow marginal tissue recession. *Journal of Periodontology* 60, 316–319.

Castellanos, A., de la Rosa, M., de la Garza, M., & Caffesse, R.G. (2006) Enamel matrix derivative and coronal flaps to cover marginal tissue recessions. *Journal of Periodontology* 77, 7–14.

Cueva, M.A., Boltchi, F.E., Hallmon, W.W., Nunn, M.E., Rivera-Hidalgo, F., & Rees, T. (2004) A comparative study of coronally advanced flaps with and without the addition of enamel matrix derivative in the treatment of marginal tissue recession. *Journal of Periodontology* 75(7), 949–956.

Gestrelius, S., Andersson, C., Johansson, A.C., Persson, E., Brodin, A., Rydhag, L., & Hammarström, L. (1997a) Formulation of enamel matrix derivative surface coating. Kinetics and cell colonization. *Journal of Clinical Periodontology* 24, 678–684.

Gestrelius, S., Andersson, C., Lidström, D., Hammarström, L., & Sommerman, M. (1997b) In vitro studies on periodontal ligament cells and enamel matrix derivative. *Journal of Clinical Periodontology* 24, 685–692.

Haase, H.R., & Bartold, P.M. (2001). Enamel matrix derivative induces matrix synthesis by cultured human periodontal fibroblast cells. *Journal of Periodontology* 72, 341–348.

Hatakeyama, Y., Uzel, M.I., Santana, R.B., & Ruben, M.P. (2005) The relationship between the position of the probe tip and periodontal tissues after periodontal surgery in dogs. *The International Journal of Periodontics & Restorative Dentistry* 25, 247–255.

Hoang, A.M., Klebe, R.J., Steffensen, B., Ryu, O.H., Simmer, J.P., & Cochran, D.L. (2002) Amelogenin is a cell adhesion protein. *Journal of Dental Research* 81, 497–500.

Jiang, J., Safavi, K.E., Spangberg, L.S., & Zhu, Q. (2001) Enamel matrix derivative prolongs primary osteoblast growth. *Journal of Endodontics* 27, 110–112.

Kalpidis, C.D.R., & Ruben, M.P. (2002) Treatment of intrabony periodontal defects with enamel matrix derivative: a literature review. *Journal of Periodontology* 73, 1360–1376.

Kawase, T., Okuda, K., Momose, M., Kato, Y., Yoshie, H., & Burns, D.M. (2001) Enamel matrix derivative (EMDOGAIN®) rapidly stimulates phosphorylation of the MAP kinase family and nuclear accumulation of smad2 in both oral epithelial and fibroblastic human cells. *Journal of Periodontal Research* 36, 367–376.

Lyngstadaas, S.P., Lundberg, E., Ekdahl, H., Andersson, C., & Gestrelius, S. (2001) Autocrine growth factors in human periodontal ligament cells cultured on enamel matrix derivative. *Journal of Clinical Periodontology* 28, 181–188.

McGuire, M.K., & Cochran, D.L. (2003) Evaluation of human recession defects treated with coronally advanced flaps and either enamel matrix derivative or connective tissue. Part 2: Histological evaluation. *Journal of Periodontology* 74, 1126–1135.

McGuire, M.K., & Nunn, M. (2003) Evaluation of human recession defects treated with coronally advanced flaps and either enamel matrix derivative or connective tissue. Part 1: Comparison of clinical parameters. *Journal of Periodontology* 74, 1110–1125.

McGuire, M.K., Scheyer, E.T., & Nunn, M. (2012) Evaluation of human recession defects treated with coronally advanced flaps and either enamel matrix derivative or connective tissue: comparison of clinical parameters at 10 years. *Journal of Periodontology* 83, 1353–1362.

Moses, O., Artzi, Z., Sculean, A., Tal, H., Kozlovsky, A., Romanos, G.E., & Nemcovsky, C.E. (2006) Comparative study of two root coverage procedures: a 24-month follow-up multicenter study. *Journal of Periodontology* 77(2), 195–202.

Ohyama, M., Suzuki, N., Yamaguchi, Y., Maeno, M., & Otsuka, K. (2002) Effect of enamel matrix derivative on the differentiation of C2C12 cells. *Journal of Periodontology* 73, 543–550.

Schwartz, Z., Carnes, D.L.J., Pulliam, R., Lohmann, C.H., Sylvia, V.L., Liu, Y., Dean, D.D., Cochran, D.L., & Boyan, B.D. (2000) Porcine fetal enamel matrix derivative stimulates proliferation but not differentiation of pre-osteoblastic 2T9 cells, inhibits proliferation and stimulates differentiation of osteoblast-like MG63 cells, and increases proliferation and differentiation of normal human osteoblast NHOst cells. *Journal of Periodontology* 71, 1287–1296.

Sculean, A., Widisch, P., Keglevich Fabi, B., Lundgren, E., & Lyngstadaas, P.S. (2002) Presence of an enamel matrix protein derivative on human teeth following periodontal surgery. *Clinical Oral Investigations* 6, 183–187.

Spahr, A., Haegewald, S., Tsoulfidou, F., Rompola, E., Heijl, L., Berni- moulin, J.P., Ring, C., Sander, S., & Haller, B. (2005) Coverage of Miller class I and II recession defects using enamel matrix proteins versus coronally advanced flap technique: a 2-year report. *Journal of Periodontology* 76(11), 1871–1880.

Tokiyasu, Y., Takata, T., Saygin, E., & Somerman, M. (2000) Enamel fac- tors regulate expression of genes associated with cementoblasts. *Journal of Periodontology* 71, 1829–1839.

van der Paw, M.T., van den Bos, T., Everts, V., & Beertsch, W. (2000) Enamel matrix-derived protein stimulates attachment of periodontal ligament fibroblasts and enhances alkaline phosphatase activity and transforming growth factor b1 release of periodontal ligament and gin- gival fibroblasts. *Journal of Periodontology* 71, 31–43.

Venezia, E., Golstein, M., Boyan, B.D., & Schartz, Z. (2004) The use of enamel matrix derivative in the treatment of periodontal defects: a literature review and meta-analysis. *Critical Reviews in Oral Biology & Medicine* 15(6), 382–402.

Zucchelli, G., & de Sanctis, M. (2000) Treatment of multiple recession- type defects in patients with esthetic demands. *Journal of Periodon- tology* 71, 1506–1514.

Chapter 11 Guided Tissue Regeneration

Serge Dibart

HISTORY

Guided tissue regeneration (GTR) is defined by the American Academy of Periodontology as a procedure attempting to regenerate lost periodontal structures through differential tissue responses (American Academy of Periodontology 1996). It involves the use of resorbable or nonresorbable barriers (membranes) to exclude epithelial and connective tissue cells from the root surface during wound healing. This is believed to facilitate the regeneration of lost cementum, periodontal ligament, and alveolar bone. In theory, this technique should result in reconstructing the attachment apparatus rather than just root coverage.

The membranes used during this procedure are most commonly made of materials such as expanded polytetrafluoroethylene (ePTFE), polyglactic acid, polylactic acid, and collagen. Pini-Prato et al. (1992) and Tinti & Vincenzi (1994) reported the use of an ePTFE membrane to treat gingival recessions. Cortellini et al. (1993) conducted a histological study on a patient, demonstrating that the root coverage obtained with the use of an ePTFE membrane, while treating a gingival recession, led to new connective tissue attachment and new bone formation. In 2001, Harris, while examining the histology of four teeth with gingival recessions treated with GTR, reported healing with a long junctional epithelium attachment without regeneration.

INDICATIONS

- Moderate to severe gingival recessions
- Thin palate
- Patient reluctant to have a second surgery site

ARMAMENTARIUM

This includes the basic surgical kit plus the following:

- Barrier membrane: resorbable (e.g., Resolut (W.L. Gore, Flagstaff, AZ, USA) XT, XTN2, or XTW1 and/or nonresorbable (e.g., Gore-Tex titanium reinforced TRN2, TRW2 or GTN1, GTN2, GTW1, or GTW2))

- Citric acid, pH 1 (40%), or 1 capsule of tetracycline hydrochloride (HCl), 250 mg

GUIDED TISSUE REGENERATION FOR ROOT COVERAGE

Technique

After proper anesthesia (Fig. 11.1), the recession is root planned thoroughly and flattened using a Gracey (Hu-Friedy, Chicago, IL, USA) curette or a back-action chisel (Fig. 11.2). The root is conditioned for 5 min with tetracycline paste. Two vertical releasing incisions are made at the line angles of the tooth with the recession (Fig. 11.3). These releasing incisions must pass the mucogingival junction for the flap to be mobile.

An intrasulcular incision connects the two verticals coronally. A full-thickness flap is raised using a periosteal elevator (24G) (Hu-Friedy) that will enable bone visibility 3 mm apical to the exposed root (Fig. 11.4). The flap is then converted to a partial thickness one apically that will enable coronal mobilization.

At this stage, the buccal flap, full at the top and partial at the bottom, when moved coronally should be able to cover and lie passively on the recession. This is critical because any tension while suturing will affect the positive outcome of the procedure. The papillae are de-epithelialized, and the membrane is trimmed and adjusted to cover the recession (Fig. 11.5).

The membrane should extend approximately 2 mm beyond the borders of the recession mesially, distally, and apically. The membrane should be coronally placed at the level of the cemento-enamel junction and sutured in place with a circumferential suture and a palatally tied knot (Fig. 11.6).

The knot is then palatally tucked into the gingival sulcus. When the sulcus is shallow, a small intrasulcular incision will help deepen it. Once the membrane is secured, the buccal flap is coronally moved and secured to the papillae with interrupted sutures (Fig. 11.7). The releasing incisions are secured with single interrupted sutures, or with figure-eight sutures on both sides. It is important, whenever possible, to not leave the membrane exposed. To avoid this, the buccal flap is usually placed

Practical Periodontal Plastic Surgery, Second Edition. Edited by Serge Dibart.
© 2017 John Wiley & Sons, Inc. Published 2017 by John Wiley & Sons, Inc.

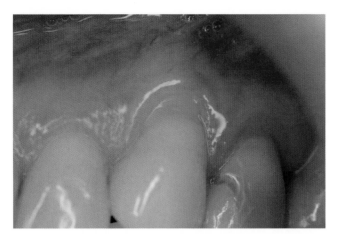

Figure 11.1 Tooth 11 with a moderate gingival recession.

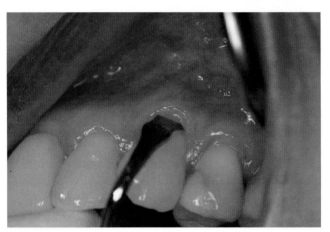

Figure 11.2 The exposed root surface is thoroughly scaled with a backaction chisel.

0.5–1.0 mm coronal to the cemento-enamel junction to cover the underlying membrane.

A periodontal dressing is then applied on the wound and left for 1 week. It is advantageous to use a resorbable membrane

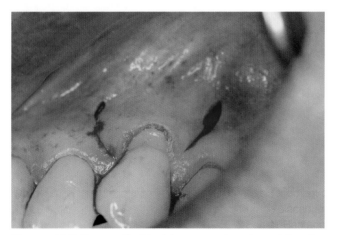

Figure 11.3 Two vertical incisions are placed, avoiding the interproximal papillae.

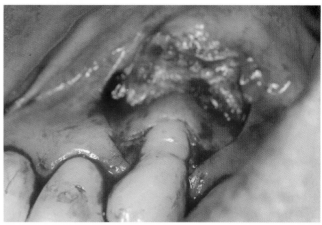

Figure 11.4 The flap is reflected, exposing some of the alveolar bone.

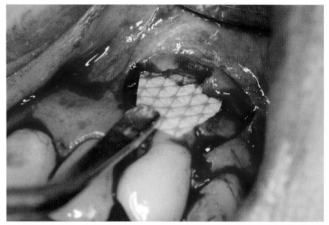

Figure 11.5 Trimming the reabsorbable membrane (Resolut) and adjusting it to fit the site.

with resorbable sutures when performing this procedure. Using a resorbable membrane with resorbable sutures eliminates the need for a second surgery, which usually follows 6 weeks later to remove the membrane. The area will heal uneventfully with

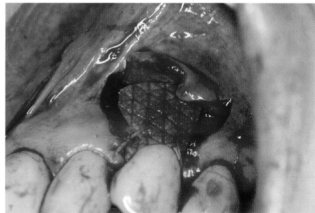

Figure 11.6 The membrane (Resolut) is secured in place with resorbable sutures.

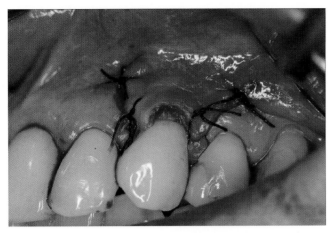

Figure 11.7 The buccal flap is sutured with the aim of covering as much of the membrane as possible.

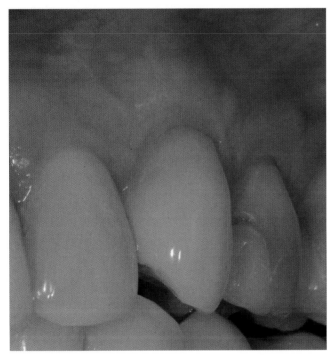

Figure 11.8 By 2 years after surgery, there is 100% coverage of the root surface.

predictable results as long as the flap was sutured tension free (Fig. 11.8).

Wound Healing

Teflon/ePTFE Membranes

These are nonresorbable, biocompatible membranes that require a second surgery for removal. There are two parts to this membrane. The first is an open microstructure collar inhibiting epithelial migration, and the second is an occlusive apron isolating the root surface from the surrounding tissues (Gottlow et al. 1986).

Polylactic Acid Membranes

These are biodegradable membranes degraded by hydrolysis. They do not require a second surgery for removal (Magnusson et al. 1988). The matrix barrier has an external layer and an internal layer separated by a space that will enable gingival connective tissue integration while excluding the epithelium (Gottlow et al. 1994).

The histology of one case (Cortellini et al. 1993) showed 3.66 mm of new connective tissue attachment, associated with 2.48 mm of new cementum and 1.84 mm of bone growth.

Possible Complications

The most common complication is membrane exposure (Fig. 11.9). If the membrane is resorbable, and there are no signs of infection, the patient should be advised to rinse with chlorhexidine gluconate. With time, the membrane will disintegrate.

If the membrane is nonresorbable and the exposure limited, the patient is given a course of antibiotics (i.e., amoxicillin, 1.5 g/day for 7 days) and asked to rinse with chlorhexidine gluconate until removal of the membrane (after 6 weeks). An infected nonresorbable membrane should be removed (Nowzari et al. 1995).

Another complication is the perforation of the flap because of the inappropriate trimming of the membrane. This occurs if the membrane is stiff and the trimming has left sharp edges. It is important when trimming the membrane to have round angles to decrease the chances of flap perforation. If the membrane is exposed, treat it in the manner already outlined.

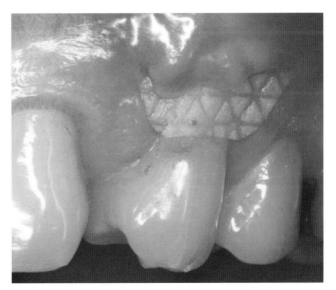

Figure 11.9 Membrane exposure 2 weeks after the surgery.

REFERENCES

American Academy of Periodontology (1996) *Annals of Periodontology World Workshop in Periodontics*. Chicago: American Academy of Periodontology, 1: 621.

Cortellini, P., Clauser, C., & Pini-Prato, G. (1993) Histologic assessment of new attachment following the treatment of a human buccal recession by means of a guided tissue regeneration procedure. *Journal of Periodontology* 64, 387–391.

Gottlow, J., Nyman, S., Lindhe, J., Karring, T., & Wennstrom, J. (1986) New attachment formation in the human periodontium by guided tissue regeneration: Case reports. *Journal of Clinical Periodontology* 13, 604–616.

Gottlow, J., Laurell, L., Lundgren, D., Mathisen, T., Nyman, S., Rylander, H., & Bogentoft, C. (1994) Periodontal tissue response to a new bioresorbable guided tissue regeneration device: A longitudinal study in monkeys. *International Journal of Periodontics and Restorative Dentistry* 14, 437–450.

Harris, R.J. (2001) Histologic evaluation of root coverage obtained with GTR in humans: A case report. *International Journal of Periodontics and Restorative Dentistry* 21, 240–251.

Magnusson, I., Batich, C., & Collins, B.R. (1988) New attachment formation following controlled tissue regeneration using biodegradable membranes. *Journal of Periodontology* 59, 1–6.

Nowzari, H., Matian, F., & Slots, J. (1995) Periodontal pathogens on polytetrafluoroethylene membrane for guided tissue regeneration inhibit healing. *Journal of Clinical Periodontology* 22, 469–474.

Pini-Prato, G., Tinti, C., Vincenzi, G., Magnani, C., Cortellini, P., & Clauser, C. (1992) Guided tissue regeneration versus mucogingival surgery in the treatment of human buccal gingival recession. *Journal of Periodontology* 63, 919–928.

Tinti, C., & Vincenzi, G.P. (1994) Expended polytetrafluoroethylene titanium reinforced membranes for regeneration of mucogingival recession defects: A 12-case report. *Journal of Periodontology* 65, 1088–1094.

Chapter 12 Acellular Dermal Matrix Graft (AlloDerm)

Serge Dibart

HISTORY

Acellular dermal matrix allograft, originally intended to cover burn wounds (Wainwright 1995), has been introduced as a less invasive alternative to soft tissue grafting (Silverstein & Callan 1997). This allograft is a freeze-dried, cellfree, dermal matrix composed of a structurally integrated basement-membrane complex and extracellular matrix in which collagen bundles and elastic fibers are the main components (Wei et al. 2000).

INDICATIONS

- Soft tissue augmentation
- Multiple adjacent gingival recessions
- Lack of graftable palatal tissue
- Patient reluctant to have a second surgical site
- Correction of gingival/mucosal amalgam tattoos

ARMAMENTARIUM

This includes the basic surgical kit, AlloDerm, sterile saline, and two sterile dishes.

TECHNIQUE

After scaling and root planning, the root surfaces are conditioned. A partial thickness flap creating a pouch is formed using a no. 15 blade (Figs. 12.1 & 12.2). All these steps are similar to those described for the subepithelial connective tissue graft.

The AlloDerm is rehydrated in two consecutive 10- to 15-min sterile saline baths (depending on size and thickness of the piece used). The graft is inserted into the pouch with the connective tissue side—the bloody side—against the recipient bed. The papillae are de-epithelialized, and the graft is immobilized with resorbable sutures at the level of the cemento-enamel junction (Fig. 12.3). The buccal flap is then sutured over the AlloDerm to cover the graft as much as possible. It is important to not leave any AlloDerm exposed, if possible (Fig. 12.4).

POSTOPERATIVE INSTRUCTIONS

Postoperative instructions include systemic antibiotherapy for 7 days after the surgery. This is helpful to avoid complications. Nonsteroidal or steroidal anti-inflammatory drugs should be prescribed to keep the pain and swelling down (Greenwell et al. 2004).

GRAFT HEALING

Significant revascularization occurs in just over 1 week. AlloDerm is repopulated with cells and will begin remodeling into the patient's own tissue over the next 3–6 months. Up to 41% shrinkage of the graft has been reported during that period (Batista et al. 2001). The material will also take the characteristics of the underlying and surrounding tissues (e.g., keratinized tissue or mucosa). Do not be concerned by the whitishness of the graft after surgery; it is not tissue necrosis. This color reflects normal healing (Fig. 12.5).

The final results are seen 2–3 years later (Fig. 12.6), sometimes with the help of a creeping attachment. It is important to remember that, when evaluating the results, the concept of gain of attached gingiva or keratinized gingiva is replaced by gain of gingival volume. The absence of keratinized tissue with this technique after successful root coverage is not uncommon, nor detrimental to the results.

REMOVAL AND CORRECTION OF AMALGAM TATTOO

The tattooed area is excised and the recipient bed prepared, as though for a free gingival graft procedure. The possible remnants of embedded amalgam particles are carefully removed from the underlying tissues, and one piece of AlloDerm is cut to size and adapted to the site. The AlloDerm is sutured

Practical Periodontal Plastic Surgery, Second Edition. Edited by Serge Dibart.
© 2017 John Wiley & Sons, Inc. Published 2017 by John Wiley & Sons, Inc.

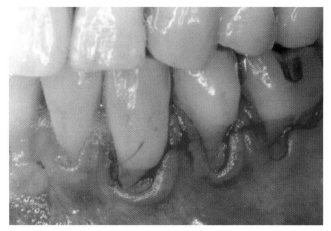

Figure 12.1 Envelope incision: a pouch is created.

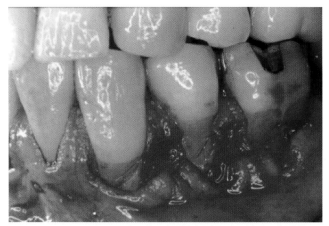

Figure 12.2 The roots are scaled, and the pouch is ready to accommodate the graft.

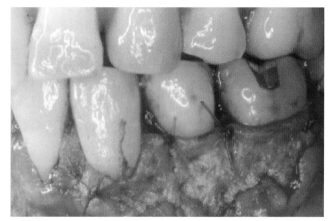

Figure 12.3 The AlloDerm is trimmed to fit the pouch, cover the roots, and suture to the papillae. These have been de-epithelialized.

carefully to the gingival margins, and a few crisscross sutures are added to immobilize the AlloDerm and prevent exfoliation. The area is then covered with a periodontal dressing (Figs. 12.7–12.10).

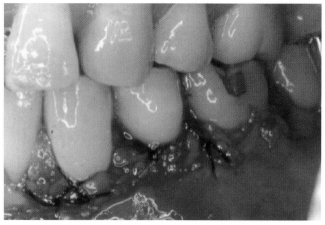

Figure 12.4 The buccal flap is sutured over the AlloDerm by using a sling suture to provide the graft with maximum coverage; 100% coverage is ideal.

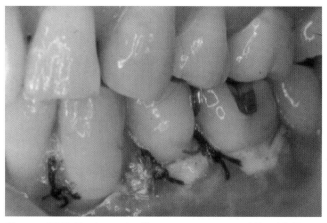

Figure 12.5 By 1 week after surgery, some of the AlloDerm is exposed. The whitishness is a normal feature of this healing process.

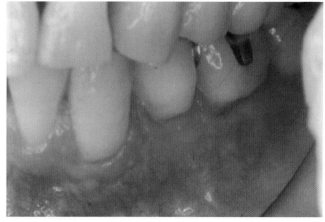

Figure 12.6 By 3 years after surgery, the recessions have been covered.

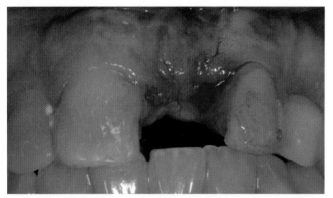

Figure 12.7 Amalgam tattoo on the gingiva, in the aesthetic zone.

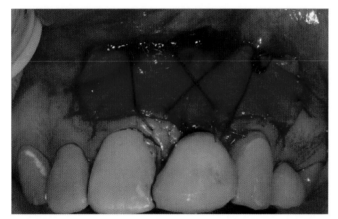

Figure 12.8 Amalgam tattoo excised and AlloDerm grafted and sutured.

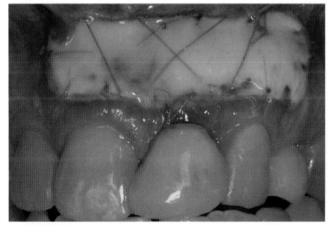

Figure 12.9 Results 1 week after surgery.

GINGIVAL GRAFTING TO INCREASE SOFT TISSUE VOLUME

For gingival grafting to increase soft tissue volume, apply the aforementioned technique, with the exception of the bed (prepared directly below the mucogingival junction) (Figs. 12.11–12.13). Shrinkage of the graft is inevitable, so plan accordingly.

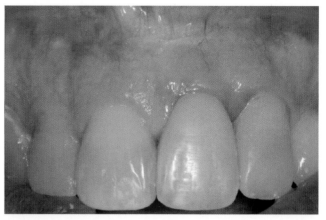

Figure 12.10 Results 1 year after surgery. The mucogingival problem has been corrected and the final prosthesis inserted.

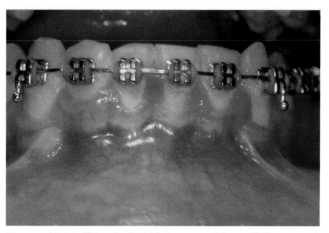

Figure 12.11 Thin gingival biotype requiring soft tissue augmentation in conjunction with orthodontic treatment.

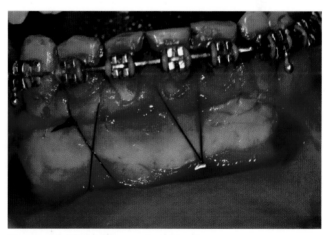

Figure 12.12 AlloDerm sutured in place.

POSSIBLE COMPLICATIONS

A possible complication of the procedure is the exfoliation of the AlloDerm if it is not well secured. AlloDerm tends to swell during the week after surgery. Another complication is infection

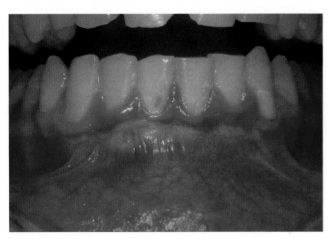

Figure 12.13 Healing of the graft at 1 year.

of the graft, necessitating its removal. Having the patient take antibiotics the day before surgery can prevent this. The patient can also be given anti-inflammatory drugs (steroidal and nonsteroidal) to control postoperative swelling and pain (Greenwell et al. 2004). This is particularly useful when using AlloDerm in ridge augmentation in edentulous areas (see Chapter 14).

REFERENCES

Batista, E.L., Batista, F.C., & Novaes, A.B. (2001) Management of soft tissue ridge deformities with acellular dermal matrix: Clinical approach and outcome after 6 months of treatment [Case series]. *Journal of Periodontology* 72(2), 265–273.

Greenwell, H., Vance, G., Munninger, B., & Johnston, H. (2004) Superficial-layer split-thickness flap for maximal flap release and coronal positioning: A surgical technique. *International Journal of Periodontics and Restorative Dentistry* 24, 521–527.

Silverstein, L.H., & Callan, D.P. (1997) An acellular dermal matrix allograft substitute for palatal donor tissue. *Postgraduate Dentistry* 3, 14–21.

Wainwright, D.J. (1995) Use of an acellular allograft dermal matrix (AlloDerm) in the management of full-thickness burns. *Burns* 21, 243–248.

Wei, P.C., Laurell, L., Geivelis, M., Lingen, M.W., & Maddalozzo, D. (2000) Acellular dermal matrix allografts to achieve increased attached gingiva. Part 1. A clinical study. *Journal of Periodontology* 71, 1297–1305.

Chapter 13 Labial Frenectomy Alone or in Combination with a Free Gingival Autograft

Serge Dibart and Mamdouh Karima

HISTORY

Frena, which are triangle-shaped folds found in the maxillary and mandibular alveolar mucosa, are located between the central incisors and canine premolar area. Frena may be long and thin, or short and broad. Labial frenum attachments have been described as mucosal, gingival, papillary, and papilla penetrating (Placek et al. 1974a & b).

Insertion points of the frena may become a problem when the gingival margin is involved (Corn 1964). This may be the result of an unusually high insertion of the frenum or marginal recession of the gingiva. High frenal insertion can distend and pull the marginal gingiva or papilla away from the tooth when the lip is stretched. This condition may be conducive to plaque accumulation and inhibit proper oral hygiene.

Aberrant frena can be treated by frenectomy or frenotomy procedures. The terms *frenectomy* and *frenotomy* signify operations that differ in degree of surgical approach. *Frenectomy* is a complete removal of the frenum, including its attachment to the underlying bone, and may be required for correction of abnormal diastema between maxillary central incisors (Friedman 1957). *Frenotomy* is the incision and relocation of the frenal attachment.

Abnormal frenal attachments occur most often on the facial surface between the maxillary and mandibular central incisors and in the canine and premolar areas (Whinston 1956). High frenal attachments on the lingual surface are less common. Orthodontic closure of diastema without excision of the associated frena are clinically associated with relapse separation of the teeth (Edwards 1977).

A frenectomy is a simple surgical procedure that can be performed separately (i.e., for orthodontic reasons) or in conjunction with a free gingival graft (i.e., to treat a gingival recession, increase the amount of attached gingival, or deepen the vestibule).

INDICATIONS

- Eliminate tension on the gingival margin (frenum-pull concomitant with or without gingival recession)
- Facilitate orthodontic treatment
- Facilitate home care

ARMAMENTARIUM

This includes the basic kit plus a mosquito hemostat.

TECHNIQUE

Surgical Steps for Frenum Removal

Grasp the frenum (Fig. 13.1) with a slightly curved hemostat inserted into the depth of the vestibule. Incise along the upper surface of the hemostat, extending beyond the tip. Make a similar incision along the undersurface of the hemostat until the hemostat is free.

Remove the triangular resected portion of the frenum with the hemostat. This exposes the underlying brushlike fibrous attachment to the bone (Fig. 13.2). Use the curved scissor to remove any dense fibers from the wound. Extend the lip and determine whether there is still pull on the periosteum. Clean the field of operation and pack it with wet gauze until bleeding subsides.

Suturing Technique

Suture the edges of the diamond-shaped wound together by using 5-0 silk in simple interrupted fashion (Fig. 13.3). Place three sutures across the wound margin to reduce postoperative discomfort and promote healing. Then apply the periodontal dressing to protect the surgical field.

Practical Periodontal Plastic Surgery, Second Edition. Edited by Serge Dibart.
© 2017 John Wiley & Sons, Inc. Published 2017 by John Wiley & Sons, Inc.

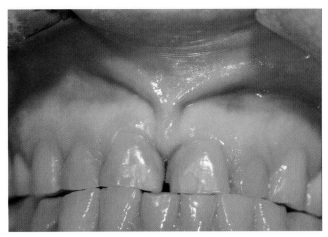

Figure 13.1 Maxillary labial frenum before frenectomy.

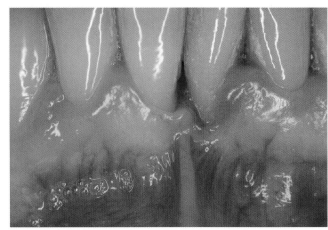

Figure 13.4 Another case of free gingival graft used to cover a buccal recession on tooth 24.

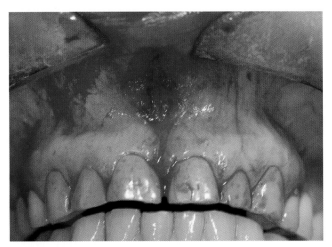

Figure 13.2 Excision of the maxillary frenum.

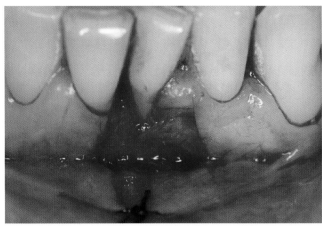

Figure 13.5 The recipient bed has been prepared, and the labial frenum excised to accommodate the gingival autograft.

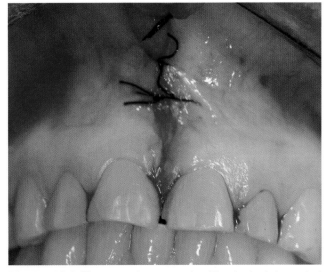

Figure 13.3 The area is secured with single interrupted sutures.

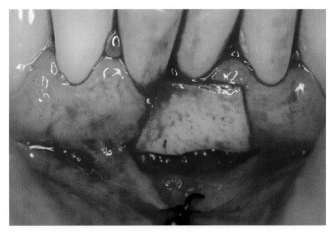

Figure 13.6 The free gingival graft is in place, with the connective tissue side against the recipient bed.

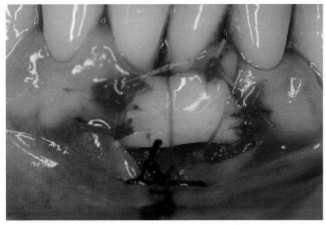

Figure 13.7 The graft is secured with resorbable 5-0 gut sutures.

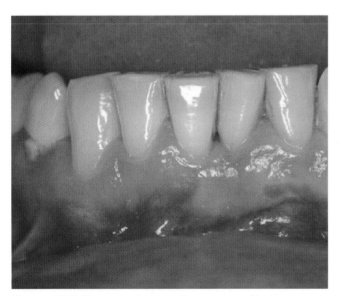

Figure 13.8 The area 1 year after surgery. Root coverage has been achieved, the amount of keratinized tissue has increased, and the frenum has been excised. Notice the restoration of the mesial papilla of tooth 24.

POSSIBLE COMPLICATIONS

Frenectomy may result in scar formation that could prevent the mesial movement of the central incisors (West 1968). However, frenectomy is typically a safe surgical procedure with no notable complications.

LABIAL FRENECTOMY IN ASSOCIATION WITH A FREE GINGIVAL AUTOGRAFT

See Figs. 13.4–13.8.

REFERENCES

Corn, H. (1964) Edentulous area pedicle grafts in mucogingival surgery. *Periodontics* 2, 229–242.

Edwards, J.G. (1977) The diastema, the frenum, the frenectomy: A clinical study. *American Journal of Orthodontics* 71, 489–508.

Friedman, N. (1957) Mucogingival surgery. *Texas Dental Journal* 75, 358–362.

Placek, M., Skach, M., & Mrklas, L. (1974a) Problems with the lip frenulum in periodontics. I. Classification and epidemiology of tendons of the lip frenulum. *Ceskoslovenska Stomatologie* 74, 385–391.

Placek, M., Skach, M., & Mrklas, L. (1974b) Problems of the labial frenum attachment in periodontics. II. Attempts to determine the resistance of periodontium to the influence of individual types of the labial frenum attachment. *Ceskoslovenska Stomatologie* 74, 401–406.

West, E. (1968) Diastema: A cause for concern. *Dental Clinics of North America* 425–434.

Whinston, G.J. (1956) Frenetomy and mucobuccal fold resection used in periodontal therapy. *New York Dental Journal* 22, 495–497.

Chapter 14 Preprosthetic Ridge Augmentation: Hard and Soft

Serge Dibart and Luigi Montesani

HISTORY

In 1983, Seibert (1983a & b) classified the different types of alveolar ridge defects that a clinician may encounter while planning a prosthetic rehabilitation. His classification described the following three clinical situations:

- Class I alveolar ridge defects have a horizontal loss of tissue with normal ridge height.

- Class II alveolar ridge defects have a vertical loss of tissue with normal ridge width.

- Class III alveolar ridge defects have a combination of class I and class II resulting in loss of normal height and width.

The reconstruction of a normal alveolar housing, in height and width, is imperative to achieve a harmonious balance between biology, function, and aesthetics.

INDICATIONS

The indications of alveolar ridge defects occur when the loss of substance compromises the positive outcome of a prosthetic restoration. This is particularly true in the aesthetic zone, and most of the time is caused by periodontal disease, careless tooth extraction, chronic infection, implant failure, congenital diseases, trauma, or neoplasm.

The loss of gingiva or bone can be detrimental to the successful placement of an implant or a fixed partial denture. This loss of substance can be avoided by socket preservation or immediate implant placement, or treated with soft and hard tissue grafting.

When planning treatment for corrective surgery, it is important to inform the patient that a single procedure may not repair the defect, so a second, or sometimes even a third, procedure is sometimes warranted. A Seibert class I defect is easier to treat than a class II, which, in turn, is easier to treat than a class III. A class III defect will require multiple grafting. In addition, the prognosis is better in the case of horizontal defects as opposed to vertical or combined defects.

These defects can be corrected by the following procedures (Table 14.1).

Soft Tissue Grafts

These are the roll technique (small to moderate class I defects), free gingival onlay grafts (class I, II, and III defects), connective tissue inlay grafts (class I defects), wedge-sandwich grafts (class I and small class II), and soft tissue allografts [AlloDerm (acellular dermal matrix allograft); LifeCell, Branchburg, NJ, USA] for class I, II, and III.

Hard Tissue Grafts

These are guided bone regeneration (GBR) with autogenous bone grafts, bone allografts, bone xenografts, synthetic bone substitutes, and block grafts.

Combination of Soft and Hard Tissue Grafts

The hard tissue graft used will depend on the extent and severity of the defect and on the type of prosthetic restoration that will follow. When an implant-supported fixed prosthesis is planned, a bone graft is needed with or without a soft tissue graft. However, when a fixed partial denture is planned, a soft tissue graft could be sufficient. It is important to keep in mind that a patient may need more than one surgery to correct a defect. In certain specific cases, procedures such as edentulous ridge expansion (ERE), distraction osteogenesis, and orthodontic treatment can be performed in conjunction with or in lieu of grafting.

ARMAMENTARIUM

This includes a basic surgical kit plus the following:

- Polytetrafluoroethylene sutures [Gore-Tex (W.L.Gore, Flagstaff, AZ, USA), suture CV-5]

- Barrier membranes: resorbable [i.e., Resolut (W.L. Gore), Bio-Gide (Osteohealth, Shirley, NY, USA), or Ossix (3i, Palm

Practical Periodontal Plastic Surgery, Second Edition. Edited by Serge Dibart.
© 2017 John Wiley & Sons, Inc. Published 2017 by John Wiley & Sons, Inc.

Table 14.1 Soft tissue versus hard tissue augmentation

Soft Tissue Grafting	Hard Tissue Grafting
Mild to moderate defects (3–6 mm)	Moderate to severe defects (>4 mm)
Horizontal defects	Horizontal and vertical defects
Fixed partial denture	Implant therapy
Availability of soft tissue	Inadequate soft tissue quantity
Questionable long-term stability	Stable with time
May need multiple augmentations	

Adapted from Pini-Prato et al. (2004).

Beach Gardens, FL, USA)] and nonresorbable [i.e., Gore-Tex expanded polytetrafluoroethylene (e-PTFE)]

- Bone allograft or substitute [i.e., Regenaform (Exactech, Gainesville, FL, USA), Dembone (Pacific Coast Tissue Bank, Los Angeles, CA, USA), Bio-Oss (Osteohealth), or Cerasorb (Curasan, Research Triangle Park, NC, USA)]

- Acellular Dermal Matrix: AlloDerm (LifeCell)

- Fixation screws: OsteoMed (Dallas, TX, USA)

- Collagen plugs: CollaPlug (Zimmer, Warsaw, IN, USA)

- Purified *n*-butyl cyanoacrylate glue (PeriAcryl) (GluStitch; Delta, BC, Canada)

SOFT TISSUE GRAFT

Technique

The soft tissue graft technique is particularly well suited when a fixed partial denture restoration is planned (Figs. 14.1 & 14.2). After proper anesthesia has been established, a partial thickness flap is elevated (Fig. 14.3). The horizontal crestal incision is slightly palatal or lingual with two vertical releasing incisions

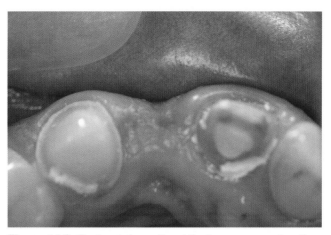

Figure 14.2 Occlusal view without the temporary restoration.

when necessary. Whenever possible, the vertical releasing incisions should be away from the external borders of the anticipated graft.

The partial thickness flap is raised and dissected beyond the mucogingival line to achieve coronal mobility. A connective tissue graft is harvested from the palate (Figs. 14.4 & 14.5), or a piece of AlloDerm is used when there is not enough autogenous tissue available. This graft is inserted under the buccal flap (Fig. 14.6) and secured to the periosteum with resorbable sutures (5-0 chromic gut P-3 needle).

The partial thickness flap is then mobilized and coronally pulled to cover the graft. Single interrupted sutures are used to close the wound by primary intention (Fig. 14.7). It is advisable to keep the sutures in place for 2 weeks to ensure enough healing of the site (Figs. 14.8–14.10).

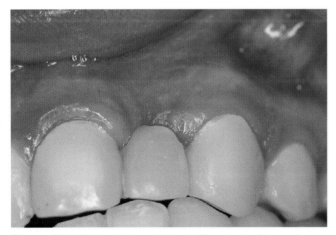

Figure 14.1 Seibert class I defect. The gingival buccal concavity needs to be augmented for a better aesthetic outcome. The restoration planned here is a fixed partial denture; hence the need for a soft tissue graft only.

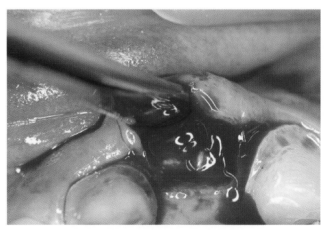

Figure 14.3 The horizontal incision is made and continued intrasulcularly to teeth 9 and 11. This helps with the sharp dissection and mobilizes the flap. An alternative would be to put two vertical incisions on each side of the area to be augmented.

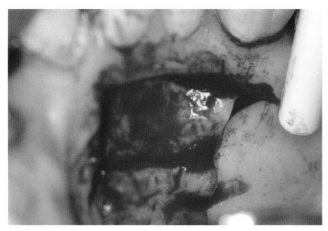

Figure 14.4 A trapdoor is opened in the palate to harvest the connective tissue graft to be used to correct the defect.

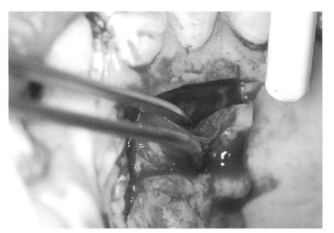

Figure 14.5 The harvest of the piece of connective tissue. The desired length and thickness have been determined by the size and shape of the defect to be corrected.

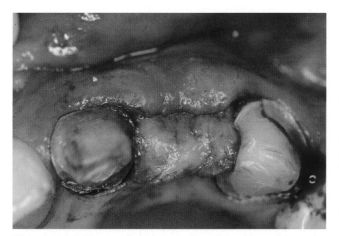

Figure 14.6 The graft is inserted and positioned into the wound. It will be secured to the periosteum bucally with an intraperiosteal horizontal mattress resorbable suture.

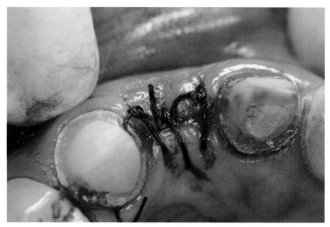

Figure 14.7 Once the connective tissue graft has been secured, the flaps are secured using single interrupted sutures.

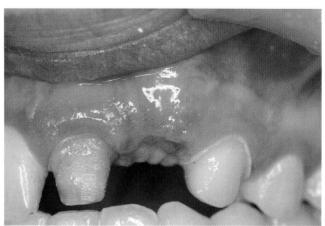

Figure 14.8 Buccal view of the augmented site 2 weeks after the surgery.

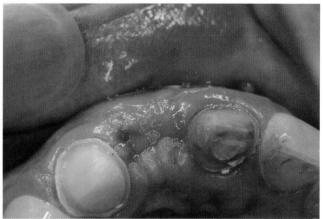

Figure 14.9 Occlusal view of the augmented site 2 weeks after the surgery. The buccal curvature has been restored.

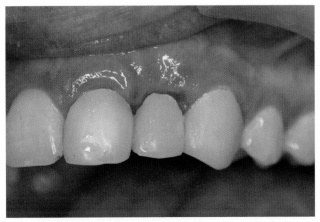

Figure 14.10 The pontic of the temporary bridge has been modified to apply light positive pressure to the area. This will help simulate papilla presence on each side of the final restoration (tooth 10).

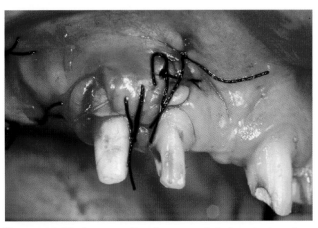

Figure 14.13 A connective tissue graft is inserted under a coronally positioned flap and secured using resorbable and silk sutures. The graft is placed on the freshly prepared root surface to re-create a zone of attached gingiva and modify the clinical crown length.

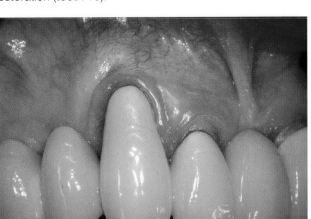

Figure 14.11 Unpleasant aesthetics as a result of iatrogenic dentistry (inadequate position of the crown margin and tooth preparation) requiring a correction of tooth 6. There is a gingival roll and inflammation around the maxillary canine and an inadequate amount of attached gingiva.

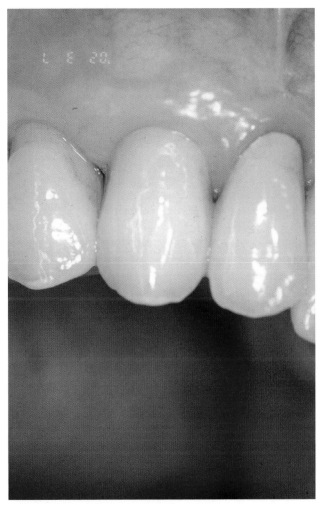

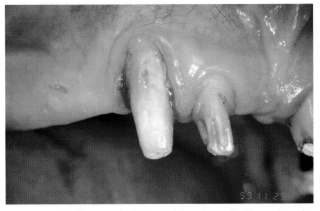

Figure 14.12 Removal of the old fixed prosthetic restoration and flattening of the exposed root and margin (rotary and hand instrumentation) in preparation for the connective tissue graft.

Figure 14.14 Final restoration 1 year later. A band of attached gingiva has been established, and pleasing aesthetics have resulted from the new position of the crown margin (tooth 6).

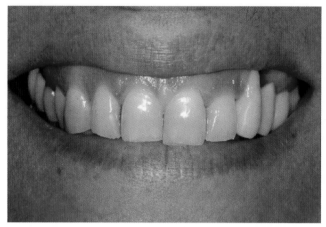

Figure 14.15 Unpleasant smile due to uneven marginal tissue height and loss of gingival volume (teeth 11 and 12).

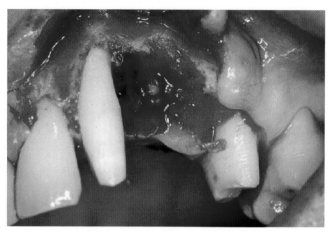

Figure 14.17 Extraction of tooth 12 and root preparation of tooth 11. Degranulation of the extraction site and preparation of the recipient bed.

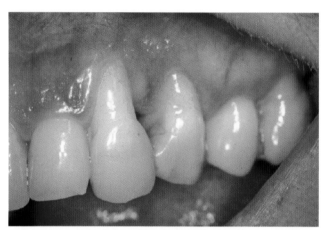

A

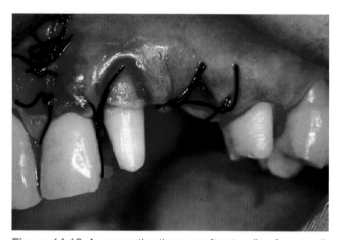

Figure 14.18 A connective tissue graft extending from tooth 10 to tooth 13 is inserted to correct the existing gingival recession on tooth 11, reestablishing a normal buccal-lingual ridge dimension.

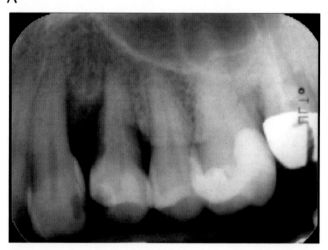

B

Figure 14.16 A: Miller class III with localized severe chronic periodontitis affecting teeth 11 and 12. **B:** Periapical radiograph of teeth 11 and 12.

CLINICAL CROWN REDUCTION USING A CONNECTIVE TISSUE GRAFT

Use this technique when the crown preparation extends too far apically with or without a lack of attached gingiva (Figs. 14.11–14.20).

HARD TISSUE GRAFT

Hard tissue grafts are primarily used when an implant-supported restoration is planned. The hard tissue augmentation can be done with block grafts (autografts and allografts), particulate grafts (cortical and cancellous), xenografts, or synthetic materials. The use of a barrier membrane is recommended with the placement of a bone graft to minimize resorption and enhance the outcome of the procedure (Antoun et al. 2001; Von Arx et al. 2001).

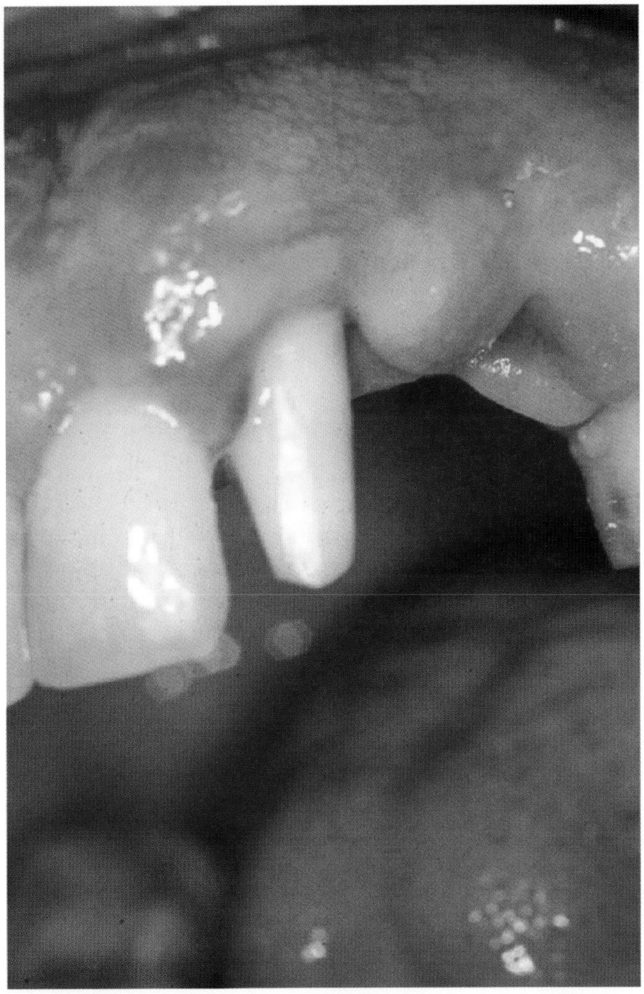

The choice of materials is usually dictated by the existing anatomy, the patient's medical history, and the size of the defect. Autogenous bone grafts, the osteogenic gold standard, have limitations, such as availability, morbidity, risk of vascular and neurological injury, and increased surgical time.

Osteoinductive allografts and osteoconductive allografts, on the other hand, are available in unlimited quantity, do not necessitate a second surgical site, have a decreased rate of patient morbidity, and shorten the time of the surgical procedure. One of their major drawbacks is the potential risk of disease transmission (Moore et al. 2001).

COMBINATION GRAFTS: HARD AND SOFT TISSUES

This is used to correct an important defect affecting the alveolar bone and soft tissue volumes (Figs. 14.21–14.39).

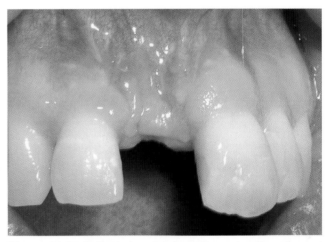

Figure 14.21 Seibert class I defect. The restoration planned here is an implant-supported crown; hence the bone tissue graft planned.

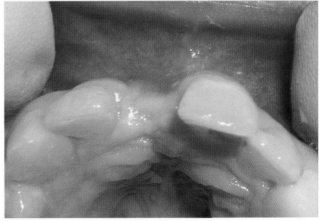

Figure 14.22 Occlusal view of the defect showing the buccal concavity that will be augmented with a bone graft.

Figure 14.19 Healing at 2 months. An interdental papilla has been created by the judicious use of the temporary prosthesis (soft tissue conditioning).

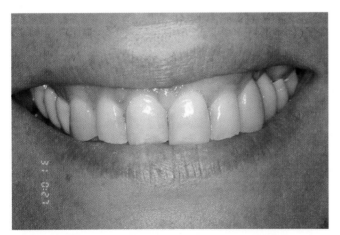

Figure 14.20 Healing at 1 year. The result is acceptable, aesthetics have improved, and the patient is satisfied.

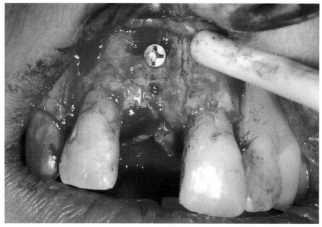

Figure 14.23 A full-thickness flap has been elevated, with a horizontal incision that is slightly palatal to the midcrest and two vertical releasing incisions. A 10-mm OsteoMed screw has been inserted halfway through the alveolar bone. This screw will serve as an anchor to the bone allograft (Regenaform) that will be placed next. The area receiving the graft has been decorticated by using a small round carbide burr.

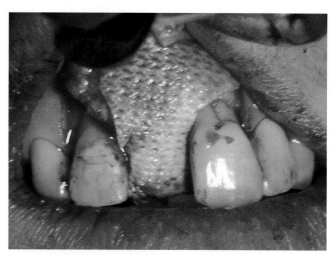

Figure 14.25 A resorbable membrane (Ossix) has been trimmed to the appropriate size and placed over the bone graft. The membrane is tucked under the palatal flap before suturing. The buccal flap is to be undermined to achieve coverage of the membrane and graft passively.

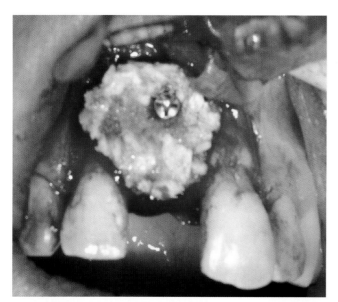

Figure 14.24 The Regenaform-block graft (10 × 10 × 5 mm), once softened, has been pushed through the screw and molded to fit the defect. When the defect is large, a second screw and a bigger graft may be necessary.

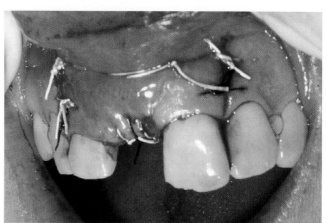

Figure 14.26 A horizontal mattress buccally and palatally with a Gore-Tex suture will hold the flaps up without tension and keep the membrane down on the bone. Additional single interrupted sutures will close the wound by primary intention.

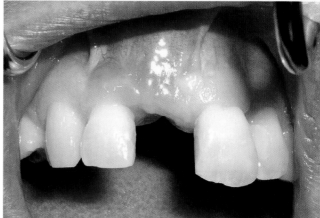

Figure 14.27 The area 1 year later. Buccal view.

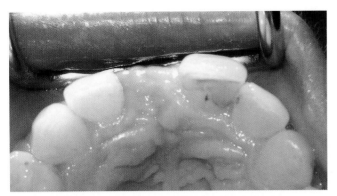

Figure 14.28 The area 1 year later. Occlusal view.

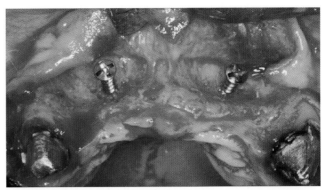

Figure 14.31 Two OsteoMed screws (1.6 × 10 mm) placed halfway into the alveolar bone.

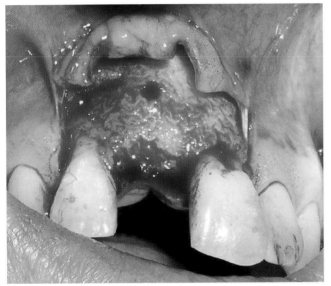

Figure 14.29 The area 1 year later at reentry and implant placement. The fixation screw was once where the red dot is.

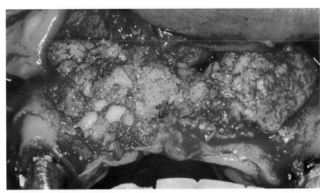

Figure 14.32 Two blocks of Regenaform (10 × 10 × 5 mm) molded and placed on the OsteoMed screws.

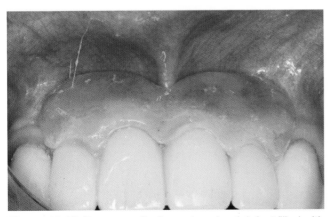

Figure 14.30 Severe vestibular and occlusal defect filled with an acrylic prosthesis to provide lip support.

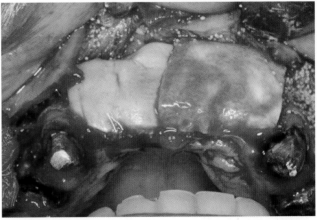

Figure 14.33 AlloDerm is used as a membrane to protect the bone graft and as a soft tissue graft to build up the vestibule. The AlloDerm is tucked under the palatal flap and secured coronally and apically to the periosteum by using resorbable sutures.

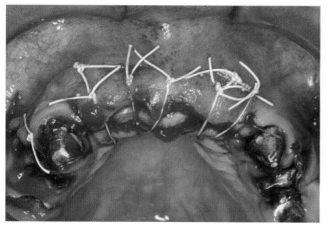

Figure 14.34 The buccal flap is coronally advanced by releasing the flap apically and secured by using horizontal mattress and single interrupted sutures (Gore-Tex). Some of the AlloDerm is left exposed, which allows for minimal coronal advancement of the flap and maintenance of the original vestibular depth.

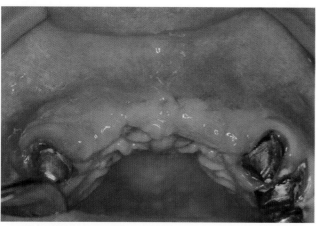

Figure 14.35 The area 3 months after the procedure.

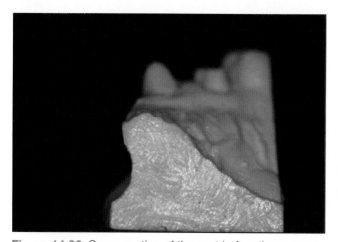

Figure 14.36 Cross-section of the cast before the surgery.

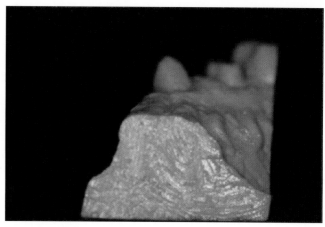

Figure 14.37 Cross-section of the cast after the surgery. Notice the amount of tissue volume gained.

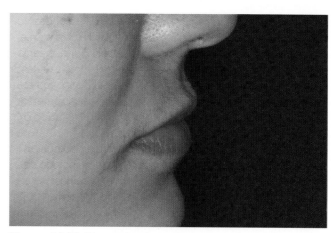

Figure 14.38 The patient's profile before the surgery. Notice the concavity of the upper lip due to the vestibular hard and soft tissue defect.

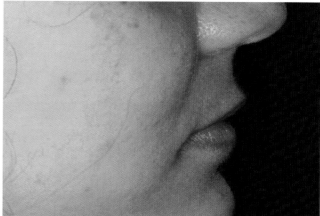

Figure 14.39 The patient's profile 3 months after surgery. Support has been provided to the upper lip, making for a better aesthetic profile.

EDENTULOUS RIDGE EXPANSION

Also known as ridge splitting, this technique is useful when there is a narrow crest, which is wider apically, with enough bone height but less than 5 mm of crestal bone width, and you plan an implant-supported prosthesis. The bone at the crest should not be all cortical because it will make this technique difficult.

The purpose of the procedure is to reposition the buccal cortical plate and increase the alveolar width by expending the edentulous ridge. In 1990, Scipioni & Bruschi introduced the bony flap in conjunction with hand chisels to expand the alveolar ridge further (Scipioni et al. 1994, 1999). In 1994, Summers introduced a ridge-expansion technique using hand osteotomes. With the right indication, this procedure enables a surgeon to place an implant in a Seibert class I defect in one session, without the need of a bone graft.

Technique

Step-by-step illustration of the ridge splitting/expansion technique allowing the placement of an implant in a Seibert class I anterior ridge defect is shown in Figs. 14.40–14.51.

SOCKET PRESERVATION

Sometimes it is necessary to extract teeth for reasons such as root fracture, periapical pathology, extensive decay, or periodontal disease. Careful removal of the tooth is completed atraumatically by using periotomes and gentle rotation movements with the forceps. Vertical and horizontal bone resorption is an inevitable natural phenomenon; there is 40% of bone height and 60% of bone width lost at 6 months (Lekovic et al. 1997, 1998).

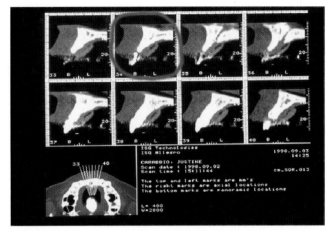

Figure 14.41 A computed-tomographic scan of the area shows a crestal bony width incompatible with successful implant placement.

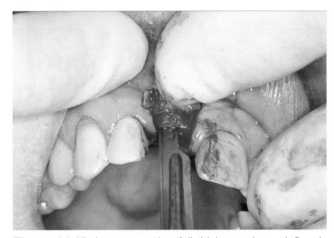

Figure 14.42 A conservative full-thickness buccal flap is raised to expose the crestal bone. Two vertical releasing incisions are placed to help mobilize the flap coronally at the end of the procedure (the flap is full thickness at the top and partial thickness at the bottom). The splitting of the ridge is initiated by using a no. 15 blade that is gently hammered in for about 5 mm.

This is further compounded by the location of the tooth to be extracted and the biotype of the patient, such as thin versus thick biotype, the former being a disadvantage. The anterior maxilla area is particularly at risk because the bone plates are thin and subject to resorption at the time of tooth removal. This can lead to the loss of bone contour and poor aesthetics. To avoid this, socket preservation becomes necessary at the time of extraction.

The Bio-Col (Bio-Oss + Collaplug) technique (Sclar 2003) or its modification helps minimize the amount of bone loss and preserve ridge aesthetics. The following technique is employed when there is no damage to the buccal plate; otherwise the use of a barrier membrane, in addition to the bone graft, becomes necessary (GBR). The rationale is that the barrier membrane

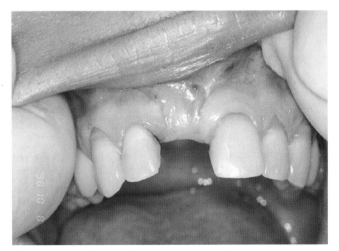

Figure 14.40 Tooth 8 is missing and will be replaced by an implant-supported crown to restore aesthetics and function.

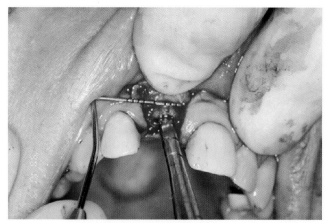

Figure 14.43 The splitting of the ridge is continued by using a bibevel osteotome chisel that will go slightly deeper than the blade and will expand the ridge to the buccal. Do not create a single large fracture. Note the minimal flap reflection.

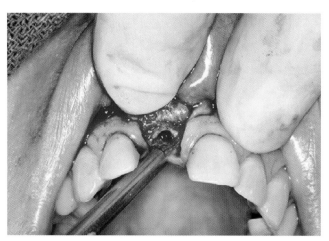

Figure 14.44 Once the midcrestal groove has been created and adequate depth obtained, the osteotomy is performed to the desired length with a 2.0-mm twist drill. This is often followed by the use of expanding osteotomes, which will condense the bone as they are expanding the osteotomy site, or proceeding with the next 3.0-mm drill.

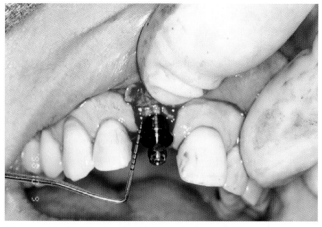

Figure 14.45 The implant is inserted carefully.

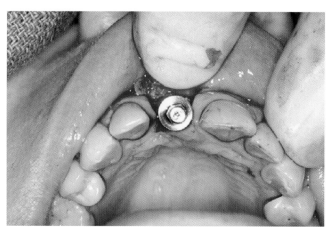

Figure 14.46 Occlusal view showing the satisfactory placement of the implant in the maxillary arch.

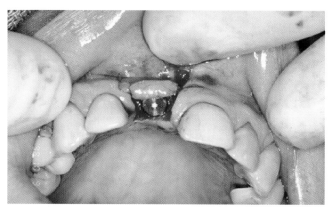

Figure 14.47 The blue mount has been removed and the cover screw tightened in place.

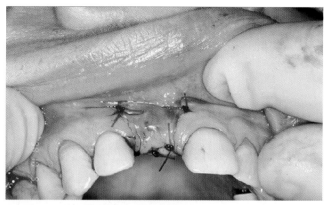

Figure 14.48 The flap is now gently advanced coronally by releasing it from the underlying periosteum (split-thickness flap) and sutured by primary intention with single interrupted sutures.

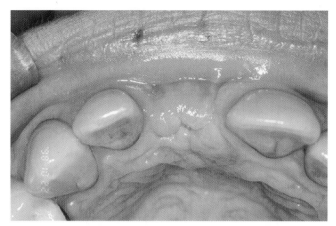

Figure 14.49 Occlusal view of the area 4 months after surgery.

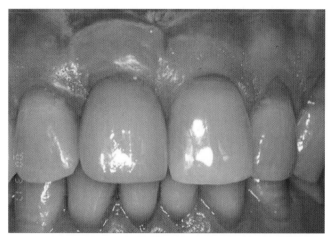

Figure 14.50 Tooth 8 is restored with an implant-supported crown. A gingival graft was needed because of gingival scars from multiple endodontic procedures.

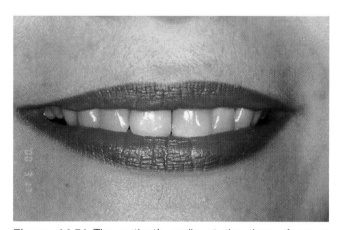

Figure 14.51 The patient's smile at the time of crown insertion.

protects the blood clot, keeps the space for new bone formation, and prevents epithelial and connective tissue cell migration to the area (Gottlow 1994). This enables the bone graft to heal undisturbed in a contained environment.

Bone that is used can be autogenous, allogenic, synthetic, or a xenograft. The only relative contraindication to this technique is active infection at the site of extraction. It is recommended to resolve the infection before grafting the socket. If a socket preservation in the presence of infection is necessary because of time constraints or other influencing factors, appropriate antibiotic treatment should be started the day before the procedure and be continued for a total of 7 days.

REFERENCES

Antoun, H., Sitbon, J.M., Martinez, H., & Missika, P. (2001) A prospective randomized study comparing two techniques of bone augmentation: Onlay graft alone or associated with a membrane. *Clinical Oral Implants Research* 12, 632–639.

Gottlow, J. (1994) Periodontal regeneration. In: Lang, N.P., & Karring, T., eds. *Proceedings of the First European Workshop on Periodontology*. London: Quintessence, 172–192.

Lekovic, V., Kenney, E.B., Weinlaender, M., Han, T., Klokkevold, P., Nedic, M., & Orsini, M. (1997) A bone regenerative approach to alveolar ridge maintenance following tooth extraction: Report of 10 cases. *Journal of Periodontology* 68, 563–570.

Lekovic, V., Camargo, P.M., KLokkevold, P.R., Weinlaender, M., Kenney, E.B., & Dimitrijevic, B. (1998) Preservation of alveolar bone in extraction sockets using bioabsorbable membranes. *Journal of Periodontology* 69, 1044–1049.

Moore, W.R., Graves, S.E., & Bain, G.I. (2001) Synthetic bone graft substitutes. *Australian & New Zealand Journal of Surgery* 71, 354–355.

Pini-Prato, G.P., Cairo, F., Tinti, C., Cortellini, P., Muzzi, L., & Mancini, E.A. (2004) Prevention of alveolar ridge deformities and reconstruction of lost anatomy: A review of surgical approaches. *International Journal of Periodontics and Restorative Dentistry* 24, 435–445.

Scipioni, A., Bruschi, G.B., & Calesini, G. (1994) The edentulous ridge expansion technique: A five-year study. *International Journal of Periodontics and Restorative Dentistry* 14, 451–459.

Scipioni, A., Bruschi, G.B., Calesini, G., Bruschi, E., & De Martino, C. (1999) Bone regeneration in the edentulous ridge expansion technique: Histologic and ultrastructural study of 20 clinical cases. *International Journal of Periodontics and Restorative Dentistry* 19, 269–277.

Sclar, A.G. (2003) Bio-Col technique for delayed implant placement. In: *Soft Tissue and Esthetic Considerations in Implant Therapy*. Carol Stream, IL: Quintessence, 75–112.

Seibert, J.S. (1983a) Reconstruction of deformed, partially edentulous ridges, using full thickness onlay grafts. Part I. Technique and wound healing. *Compendium of Continuing Education in Dentistry* 4, 437–453.

Seibert, J.S. (1983b) Reconstruction of deformed, partially edentulous ridges, using full thickness onlay grafts. Part II. Prosthetic/periodontal interrelationships. *Compendium of Continuing Education in Dentistry* 4, 549–562.

Summers, R.B. (1994) The osteotome technique. Part 2. The ridge expansion osteotomy (REO) procedure. *Compendium of Continuing Education in Dentistry* 15, 422–426.

Von Arx, T., Cochran, D.L., Herman, J.S., Schenk, R.K., & Buser, D. (2001) Lateral ridge augmentation using different bone fillers and barrier membrane application: A histologic and histomorphometric pilot study in the canine mandible. *Clinical Oral Implants Research* 12, 260–269.

Chapter 15 Exposure of Impacted Maxillary Teeth for Orthodontic Treatment

Serge Dibart and Lorenzo Montesani

HISTORY

Impactions of the maxillary teeth, canines in particular, can be classified as labial, palatal, and intermediate (Kruger 1984). Precise localization of the crown through intraoral radiographs is important to determine the surgical approach and the flap design.

INDICATION

- Exposure of impacted teeth

ARMAMENTARIUM

This includes the basic kit plus surgical round burrs (carbide or diamond). The piezotome is also very useful in conjunction with the Piezocision™ procedures aimed at accelerating the rate of tooth movement during orthodontic treatment.

TECHNIQUE

After localization of the crown, buccally or palatally, the area is anesthetized. In the case of buccal impaction, it is critical to design the incision to retain as much attached gingiva as possible to avoid a mucogingival defect afterward (Fig. 15.1). A full-thickness flap with vertical releasing incisions is elevated to expose the underlying bony bulge (Fig. 15.2).

At this point, the crown is either only partially visible or not visible. A round burr (no. 4 or no. 6) can be used to expose the crown further. The flap is then apically repositioned and sutured below the exposed crown. An apical sharp dissection may be necessary to enable flap fixation (to the periosteum). After a short healing phase (Fig. 15.3), an orthodontic bracket is secured on the crown for future tooth alignment.

In case of palatal crown location, an open or a closed approach is possible.

Open Approach

A semilunar incision is made on the palate and the crown exposed with or without ostectomy (Fig. 15.4). Since we cannot apically position the flap in the palate, a scissor is used to cut off the tip of the flap and leave the crown exposed. At this point, a bracket is placed on the crown (Fig. 15.5).

Closed Approach

In the closed approach (Fig. 15.6), there is no need to resect the palatal tissue. After careful clinical and radiographic evaluation (making sure that there is no evident signs of tooth ankylosis) (Fig. 15.7) a full-thickness palatal flap is raised to expose the impacted tooth (Fig. 15.8).

It is very important to have enough visibility and access to clear the space around the clinical crown from the residual dental sac. At this point care must be taken not to "wiggle" the tooth and resist the urge to luxate it. Bone can be removed to facilitate the path of descent. Piezocision cuts can be done simultaneously to facilitate and accelerate canine tooth movement.

The clinical crown can now be bonded with a button and a chain. Care must be taken not to spill etching or bonding agents into the periodontal ligament that is exposed. The palatal flap is then sutured back with 4 × 0 chromic gut interrupted sutures (Fig. 15.9).

The canine is brought down with conventional orthodontic mechanics (Fig. 15.10) and the case finished satisfactorily (Fig. 15.11).

Practical Periodontal Plastic Surgery, Second Edition. Edited by Serge Dibart.
© 2017 John Wiley & Sons, Inc. Published 2017 by John Wiley & Sons, Inc.

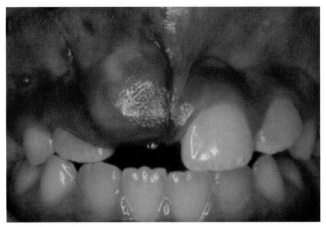

Figure 15.1 A buccal full-thickness flap is elevated to expose the crown of tooth 8.

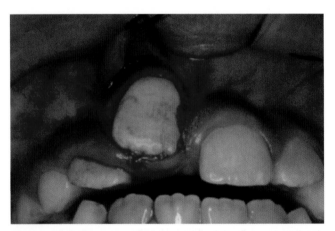

Figure 15.2 The crown is exposed and the flap sutured apically (not shown).

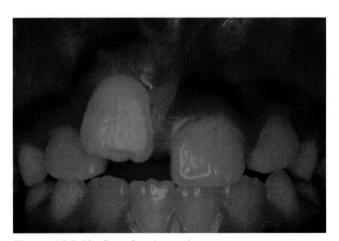

Figure 15.3 Healing after 1 month.

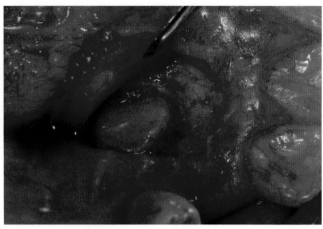

Figure 15.4 A palatal semilunar flap to expose an impacted canine.

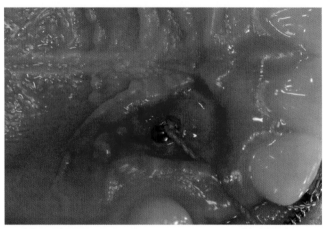

Figure 15.5 The tip of the flap has been trimmed and a bracket placed on the exposed crown.

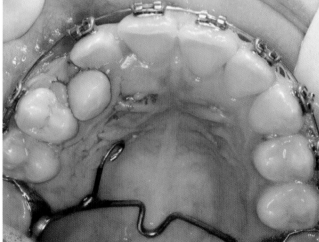

Figure 15.6 Thirteen-year-old with impacted canine (tooth 6).

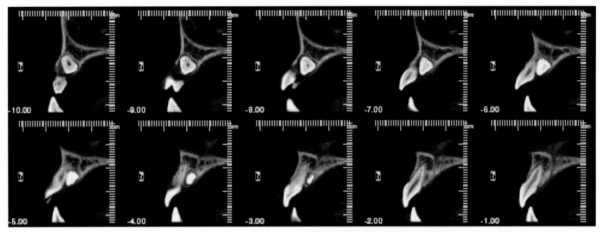

Figure 15.7 CT scan showing the level of impaction and the presence of the periodontal ligament.

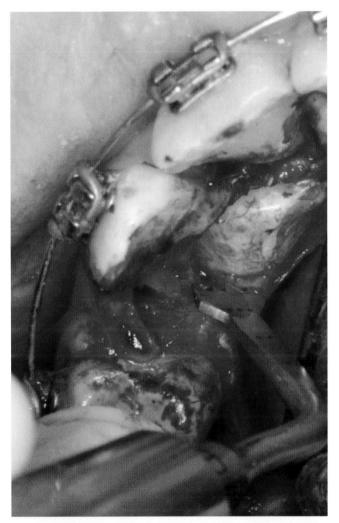

Figure 15.8 The primary canine has been extracted and a full-thickness palatal flap has been raised. The permanent canine has been exposed and the follicular sac around the clinical crown removed. Piezocision cuts are made to accelerate tooth movement.

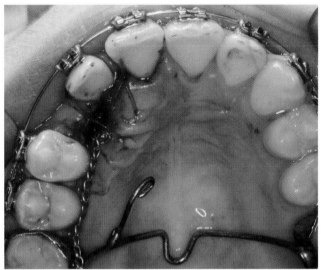

Figure 15.9 After the permanent canine has been exposed and a chain secured to the clinical crown the flap is closed using 4 × 0 chromic gut sutures.

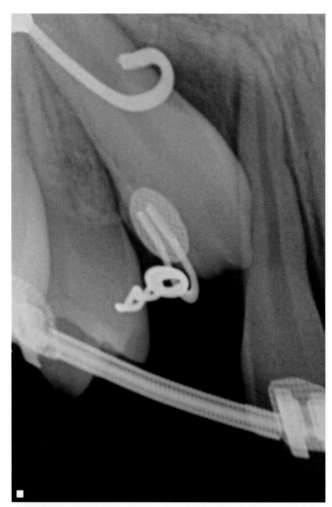

Figure 15.10 A few months later the canine is coming down through the gingiva.

REFERENCE

Kruger, G.O. (1984) *Oral and Maxillofacial Surgery*, 6th edition. St Louis: C.V. Mosby, 91–93.

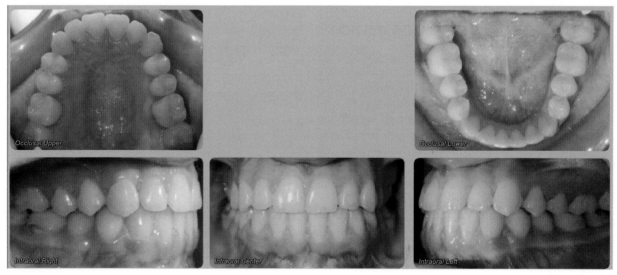

Figure 15.11 The patient has completed the treatment.

Chapter 16 Peri-implant Soft Tissue Management

D.M. Diego Capri

FOREWORD

In reviewing this chapter for the second edition of the book an attempt was made to update the bibliography by including scientifically relevant papers published over the last few years.

The hope was to be able to list recent randomized clinical trials or good-quality systematic reviews relevant to the topic of soft tissue management around dental implants to better substantiate the clinical strategies presented to the reader.

While new information was indeed available in the literature allowing us to strengthen some of the previously presented therapeutic concepts, or to divert from disproven ones, many of the controversial issues still remain.

There is a need for more and better research in the area of peri-implant soft tissue management.

INTRODUCTION

Implant therapy has significantly evolved during the last three decades from being one of the treatments of choice for edentulous arches (Adell et al. 1981) to becoming a routine procedure to replace lost dental elements, regardless of the type of edentulism. With this development the objective of implant therapy has expanded from the functional restoration of the missing dentition to include the re-creation of the lost hard and soft tissues (Garber & Belser 1995).

Only when a close resemblance with what once existed in nature is achieved does the end result of implant therapy become a success, for its ability to exert the proper masticatory function while "disappearing" in between the remaining natural teeth.

For an implant restoration to mimic closely the lost dental element, it is undoubtedly important to select the shape and color of the prosthetic tooth properly, but nonetheless it is imperative to surround the crown with healthy gingival-like tissue (Figs. 16.1–16.4).

GINGIVAL TISSUES AND PERI-IMPLANT MUCOSA

When handling the peri-implant soft tissue it is important to acknowledge the differences that exist between the peri-implant mucosa and the gingival tissue.

The mucosa that encircles the fixture presents with more collagen and fewer fibroblasts (2:1 ratio) when compared to the periodontal gingival tissue (Berglundh et al. 1991; Abrahamsson et al. 2002). The collagen fibers of the healthy periodontium are functionally arranged in a complex system (Smukler & Dreyer 1969) that differs from the fiber bundles of the peri-implant mucosa (Schierano et al. 2004), which run mostly parallel to the titanium surface without attaching to it (Berglundh et al. 1991). It has been reported that both the titanium surface characteristics (Schroeder et al. 1981; Piattelli et al. 1997; Rompen et al. 2006; Schupbach & Glauser 2007) and the mobility of the soft tissues (Listgarten et al. 1991) would affect the collagen fibers orientation. Material characteristics, surface topography, and implant components and connections have been investigated (Rompen et al. 2006) for their role in differentiating epithelial and connective tissue adhesion to the fixture. Some implant surface roughness and microgrooves may be effective in stopping the epithelial downgrowth while improving the connective tissue ingrowth. The cleanliness of transgingival abutments from contaminants seems to be relevant in avoiding detrimental effects on the soft tissues and once compromised, an attempt to decontaminate is unlikely to regain a pristine condition. (Rompen et al. 2006).

Recently canine and human histology has been presented (Nevins et al. 2008, 2010a, 2012; Iglhaut et al. 2013) regarding the possibility of attracting a physical connective tissue attachment to an implant surface, or to an abutment, using a micro-textured surface presenting with a 0.7 μm wide series of micrometric grooves. According to the authors the micro-grooved band was able, by the creation of a fibrous attachment to the implant or the abutment, to prevent the downgrowth of the junctional epithelium and, as a consequence of that, to significantly reduce/eliminate the usual amount of bone loss.

Practical Periodontal Plastic Surgery, Second Edition. Edited by Serge Dibart.
© 2017 John Wiley & Sons, Inc. Published 2017 by John Wiley & Sons, Inc.

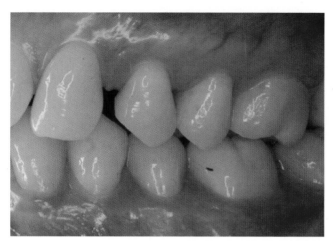

Figure 16.1 Pre-operative buccal view. The first premolar is fractured.

While acknowledging how new features in the macro- and micro topography of implants and abutments can positively alter the responses of surrounding tissues, the clinical significance of such tissue reactions still needs to be elucidated through further investigations.

The lack of a cemental layer with functionally inserted Sharpeys fibers still remains the major distinctive attribute when comparing the dentogingival junction with the implant soft tissue interface. As a consequence of this, the diverse histological characterization the gingiva surrounding the implant lacks mechanical resistance when compared to the truly attached gingiva of the natural tooth.

In other words, even when the fibers are more perpendicularly disposed there is no real functional insertion of them.

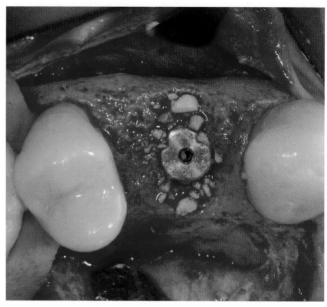

Figure 16.3 At 6 weeks after the extraction, a single implant is placed into the residual socket and a xenograft is used to fill the voids between the implant and the osseous walls.

The supracrestal vascular topography that is found surrounding the fixture is reduced and diversely arranged when compared to the supracrestal vessels of a natural dental element (Berglundh et al. 1994; Moon et al. 1999).

Research conducted on dogs has shown that both the tooth and the implant present with a junctional epithelium of approximately 2 mm in length (Berglundh et al. 1991). Human histology, albeit limited, of the peri-implant mucosa has been shown (Glauser et al. 2005) to have a total height of the soft tissue surrounding the implant of 4–4.5 mm. While the peri-implant sulcus depth varied, depending on the treatment of the implant

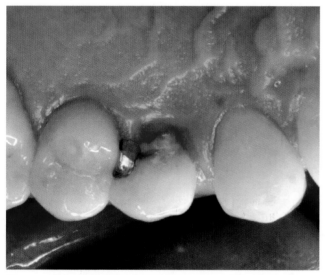

Figure 16.2 Pre-operative palatal view. The fracture line extends several millimeters subgingivally.

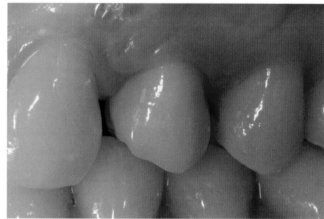

Figure 16.4 The final implant-supported restoration is in place. There is a harmonious integration of the prosthetic crown in between the natural dental elements and the healthy and natural appearance of the peri-implant gingiva.

surface, between 0.2 and 0.5 mm, the height of the junctional epithelium ranged between 1.4 and 2.9 mm, with a vertical variation for the connective tissue component between 0.7 and 2.6 mm.

The reader should be reminded how histomorphometric average values, for the highly variable epithelial junction in humans, were reported to be around 1 mm (Gargiulo et al. 1961; Vacek et al. 1994). More considerations on the dimension of the peri-implant mucosa in comparison with the marginal periodontium will follow in the section on biological width.

In spite of the clinical, almost indistinguishable, appearance between the peri-implant soft tissue and the gingiva encircling a natural dental element, the histological dissimilarities mentioned above are important in the selection of the most appropriate way to manage the implant mucosa.

The tissue that encompasses the fixture, with its lower cellularity and reduced vascularity, resembles cicatritial tissue and as such requires special care when surgically challenged. In the basic periodontal wound-healing processes, after flap elevation, one of the most dynamic tissues involved is the periodontal ligament (Goldman & Cohen 1980). The lack of this ligament with its vessels and cells must be taken into consideration by the surgeon who is conducting the peri-implant mucosa. While periodontal plastic procedures are daily used to correct peridental sites where mucogingival problems have already occurred, in implant therapy the less forgiving nature of the tissues involved makes it advisable to initially optimize the peri-implant soft tissues in order to prevent future complications. The quality and quantity of the peri-implant tissues should be improved either before or at implant placement, during the submerged healing, or at the time of second stage surgery (Nevins & Mellonig 1998; Kazor et al. 2004).

In fact some root coverage procedures should not be considered for implants in communication with the oral environment (one-stage implants, uncovered two-stage implants, or implants supporting a prosthesis) as they are around natural teeth (Harris 1994; Sclar 2003). In the attempt to cover an exposed implant–abutment complex, or to mask the grayish color that appears through a thin peri-implant mucosal tissue, surgical approaches, such as the variously displaced pedicle flaps (coronally, laterally, double papilla, etc.) or free gingival autografts, usually fall short. In such unfortunate clinical scenarios, and provided that the angle of emergence of the implant–abutment–crown complex is not excessively buccal, a coronally advanced flap augmented by a subepithelial connective tissue graft represents the most predictable procedure because of its double-blood supply (Langer & Langer 1985; Nelson 1987).

A 6-month prospective cohort study of 10 patients presenting with a soft tissue dehiscence on single implants reported how a coronally advanced flap covering a free connective tissue graft could significantly improve the clinical lesions. At the end of surgery all soft tissue recessions were completely covered with an average overcompensation of 0.5 mm, but by the end of the observation period none of the sites were completely covered.

The mean depth of recession in the study was 3 ± 0.8 mm and after 1 month the average coverage measured was equal to 75% (standard deviation (SD) 17%), a value that decreased to 70% and then to 66% (SD 18%) after 3 and 6 months, respectively.

Flap thickness was discussed as being positively correlated with the average recession coverage while initial dehiscence depth seemed to negatively affect the treatment outcomes (Burkhardt et al. 2008).

A prospective pilot study was recently published (Zucchelli et al. 2013) modifying the clinical approach previously reported by Burkhardt et al. (2008). Twenty single implants with an average soft tissue defect of 3 mm were treated and followed for 1 year with a combined surgical and prosthetic therapy.

The extremely positive results (96.3% defect coverage at 12 months and 75% of the lesions with complete resolution) were attributed to the significant pre-operative abutment reduction and new temporization of the implant, the different harvesting technique of the graft (one line incision for the 2008 study versus de-epithelization of a superficial 2-mm thick free gingival graft for the current research), and the extended removal of the epithelium occlusally and palatally in the interproximal soft tissue areas. In other words the authors obtained significantly improved results by widening the vascular recipient bed through a significant reduction in the prosthetic components that later allowed for enlargement of the surgical area toward the palate, and by improving the quality of the connective tissue graft via a different surgical procurement technique (Zucchelli et al. 2010).

Excellent stability of the grafted soft tissue was reported in terms of both vertical dehiscence coverage and horizontal soft tissue thickness increase, which was 1.5 mm on average.

In particularly difficult clinical cases, removing the prosthetic components to re-submerge the fixture can be useful to widen palatally the recipient vascular bed for the subepithelial connective tissue graft. This further increases the predictability of success.

THE NEED FOR KERATINIZED TISSUE

The need for keratinized tissue around the implant is still controversial (Adell et al. 1981; Wennstrom et al. 1994; Warrer et al. 1995). Two systematic reviews came to the conclusion that there is currently not enough reliable evidence to claim that increasing the amount of peri-implant keratinized mucosa creates any benefit for the patient (Esposito et al. 2007, 2012). In spite of this the presence of gingival-like tissue presents several important advantages. The keratinized gingival tissue provides a tight fibrous collar that surrounds the implant, sealing off the bacteria from the depth of the peri-implant sulcus (Warrer et al. 1995). A report in 1990 by Block & Kent on the beneficial effects on soft and hard tissue health of having keratinized tissue around implants examined more than 700 implants prospectively (Block & Kent 1990) A retrospective study on 32 patients examining 63 implants evaluated how keratinized mucosal width and thickness affected both clinical and immunological parameters (Zigdon & Machtei 2008). The authors reported a moderately positive correlation between the width of keratinized mucosa and probing depth, but also a negative correlation between keratinized mucosa width and mucosal recession, probing attachment level, and prostaglandin E2 levels in peri-implant crevicular fluid. A similar type of correlation was identified for mucosal thickness and probing depth (positive correlation) or mucosal recession (negative correlation). A wider peri-implant keratinized mucosal band (>1 mm) was associated with less recession and less peri-implant attachment loss when compared with implants with a narrow ($\leq$ 1 mm) band (0.27 and 0.9 mm, $P = 0.001$, and 2.65 and 3.34 mm, $P = 0.001$, respectively). When evaluating the mucosal thickness, areas with thick mucosa ($\geq$ 1 mm) presented with less recession than areas where the mucosa was less than 1 mm (0.45 and 0.9, respectively, with $P = 0.04$). The restorative maneuvers that precede crown placement are potentially detrimental to tissue health and the presence of an immobile keratinized tissue seems, at least from an immediate clinical impression, to better withstand the trauma that is caused. In the review by Rompen et al. (2006) it is stated that in order to reach the goal of improving the quality and thus stability of the implant/soft tissue interface, surgical techniques should be chosen with the aim of preserving or reconstituting a fibrous, keratinized, and stable gingiva.

The presence of keratinized mucosa seems to favor a more perpendicular orientation of the connective tissue fibers to the implant surface, which different to the parallel fiber orientation observed when the transmucosal area abuts alveolar mucosa (Rompen et al. 2006).

Plaque control in the presence of a band of keratinized mucosa is easier for the patient and for the hygienist during periodic maintenance recalls (Figs. 16.5–16.9). Two cross-sectional observations on hundreds of implants showed that implants with narrow zones of keratinized tissue (<2 mm) had significantly more plaque and signs of inflammation than those with wider zones of keratinized gingiva ($\geq$2 mm) (Chung et al. 2006; Bouri et al. 2008). While Bouri et al. found a significant independent association between the width of keratinized mucosa and

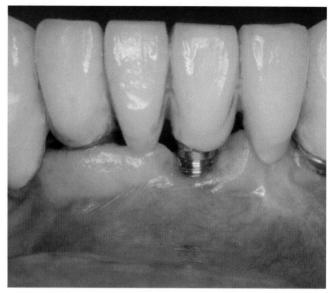

Figure 16.5 Pre-operative view. The patient, treated with an implant-supported restoration 12 years ago, now complains about discomfort during daily oral hygiene procedures.

radiographic bone loss in favor of wider areas of keratinization, Chung et al. came to the opposite conclusion. It should be remembered that the cross-sectional design of these studies is not appropriate to evaluate any relation of causality and that randomized clinical trials should be designed to confirm or

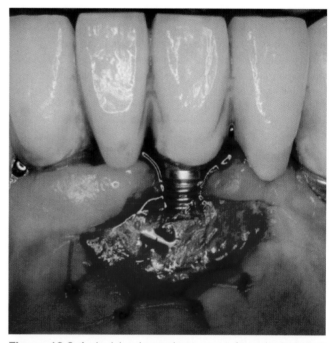

Figure 16.6 A decision is made to use a free gingival graft to increase the amount of keratinized tissue. The main goal is to simplify the home oral hygiene procedures. A periosteal bed has been prepared. There is dehiscence buccal to the otherwise osseointegrated implant.

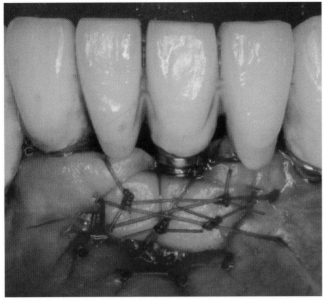

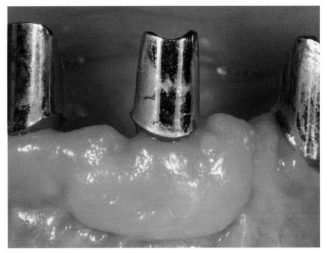

Figure 16.7 A thick, free gingival graft is carefully adapted to the periosteal bed and stabilized with compressive 5-0 gut sutures. No attempt is made to cover the original marginal recession.

Figure 16.9 After 3 years, during a periodical hygiene recall, stability of the area is evident. The creeping phenomenon progressed for an additional 0.5 mm (compare with Fig. 16.8).

disprove the above findings. The possibility that insufficient keratinization of the implant mucosa increases the risk of crestal bone loss and gingival recession was statistically confirmed in the retrospective analysis by Kim et al. (2009). The same group could not find a statistical association between deficient keratinized mucosa and adverse effects on the level of oral hygiene or gingival inflammation in a studied sample of 100 patients with 276 implants. A smaller retrospective cross-sectional

study of 66 implants supporting maxillary and mandibular overdentures found significantly less plaque accumulation, gingival inflammation, bleeding on probing, and mucosal recession when adequate keratinization of the soft tissue was present (P <0.05). A wider keratinized mucosal band ($\geq$2 mm) was associated with less recession and peri-implant attachment loss (Adibrad et al. 2009). In 2009 a 5-year prospective multi-center clinical trial evaluated the soft tissue health and stability of 307 implants, supporting full arch fixed mandibular prosthesis in 58 patients. The research concluded that in the patient population observed, regularly maintained and characterized by a good level of oral hygiene, the presence of at least 2 mm of keratinized mucosa was beneficial in reducing lingual peri-implant plaque accumulation and bleeding, as well as buccal soft tissue recession. Sites with a minimum of 2 mm of buccal keratinized tissue presented with an average recession of 0.08 mm in comparison with a mean of 0.69 mm measured in areas with less than 2 mm ($P < 0.001$) (Schrott et al. 2009). Further research on a limited number of mandibular implants (36) confirmed some of the observations previously reported in retrospective studies and came to the conclusion that an adequate band of keratinized mucosa may be related to statistically less plaque accumulation, less peri-implant mucosal inflammation, and less pro-inflammatory mediators (TNF-α) (Boynuegry et al. 2013).

A narrative review paper published in 2012 by Wennström & Derks (2012) came to the conclusion that the analyzed reported evidence, much of which came by way of reviewing some of the above-mentioned papers, only offers limited support to the need for keratinized mucosa to maintain health and tissue stability around implants. When discussing if a limited amount of keratinization influences the patient's oral hygiene measures the authors concluded that the available data do not show that an inadequate amount of keratinized tissue per se obstructs daily oral hygiene maneuvers.

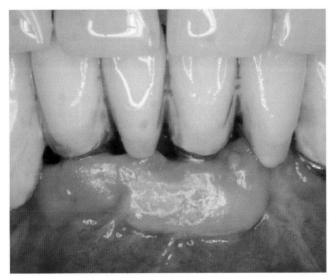

Figure 16.8 Final healing of the area. The patient did not experience any further discomfort during brushing. An unexpected creeping attachment phenomenon of about 2 mm was also obtained.

With regard to a lack of a keratinized band of mucosa and presence of soft tissue recession or bone loss around implants, Wennström & Derks (2012) highlight the paucity of well-conducted prospective clinical trials and observe how, when changes are indeed measured, they tend to happen early in the first 6–12 months post implant restoration. This phenomenon does not favor the concept that an adequate band of keratinized mucosa would be significant in the long-term maintenance of soft and hard tissue health and stability. Some surgical interventions to augment the missing keratinized mucosa might be considered, according to the same authors, for patients who experience pain or discomfort during brushing and thus present with substandard levels of oral hygiene (Wennström & Derks 2012).

Regarding per-iimplant soft tissue health and stability several authors (Pjetursson et al. 2004; Ferreira et al. 2006; Schmidlin et al. 2010) have reported a high rate of biological implant complications such as mucositis or peri-implantitis. A paper published in 2010 by Koldsland highlighted how the prevalence of peri-implantitis could vary, depending on the criteria chosen to define the disease, from a minimum of 11.3% to a maximum of 47.1% of the subjects (Koldsland et al. 2010).

With the objective of profiling the risk of developing peri-implant disease a number of factors, including the absence of keratinized tissue, were investigated in a multivariate analysis of potential explanatory variables (Roos-Jansaker et al. 2006). In this study on more than 200 patients the absence of keratinized peri-implant mucosa could not be associated with peri-implant disease.

In addition to the above-mentioned research a 2012 study followed the fate of a group of patients initially diagnosed with mucositis (Costa et al. 2012). During a period of 5 years 31.2% of the mucositis cases evolved into peri-implantitis and an absence of at least 1 mm of keratinized tissue was listed as one of several factors significantly ($P = 0.001$) associated with the evolution of the pathology.

Obtaining peri-implant tissue that resembles the keratinized gingiva present on the adjacent natural teeth becomes important in the esthetic zone (Bashutski & Wang 2007). The free autogenous gingival graft still represents the preferred procedure to predictably increase the keratinized soft tissue that encircles the implant (Sullivan & Atkins 1968; Ten Bruggenkate et al. 1991).

BIOLOGICAL WIDTH AND GINGIVAL BIOTYPES

Biological width traditionally refers to the sum of two histological peri-dental entities: the junctional epithelium and the connective tissue attachment (Gargiulo et al. 1961; Vacek et al. 1994). The importance of these two distinct, but related, tissues within the environment of the dentogingival junction has been amply debated in the literature (Maynard & Wilson 1979; Smukler & Chaibi 1997).

The integrity of the dental biological width (average histological value of 2.04 mm) protects, by its biological sealing property, the other underlying deep periodontal tissues that are kept separated from the outer oral and sulcular environment (average histological value of 0.69 mm) (Listgarten et al. 1991). Known for its high histological variability, the biological width together with the gingival sulcus concur to form the different clinical periodontal biotypes (Weisgold et al. 1997), more recently redefined as periodontal phenotypes (Muller & Eger 2002). The main and most immediate clinical expression of the periodontal biotype is related to the degree of scalloping of the gingival tissues. The outline of the gingiva and its scalloping reflects the osseous morphotype of the underlying supporting osseous crest (Becker et al. 1997). The dental anatomy, with its convexities and concavities, also affects both the soft and hard tissues, which peak in the tooth surface depressions and fall in areas of surface protuberance (Olsson et al. 1993; Smukler & Chaibi 1997).

Whereas the gingiva and the osseous crest normally run parallel to each other, and to the tooth cemento-enamel junction buccally and lingually (or palatally), in the interproximal area the position of the gingival tissues is also affected by other variables, and may or may not follow the osseous crest profile (Smukler & Chaibi 1997). Factors such as the position of the adjacent dental elements and their anatomy determine the shape and location of the contact point, and together with the interproximal peak of bone determine papillary form and height (Tarnow et al. 1992).

Under normal circumstances the height of the soft tissue column located interproximally is superior to the height of the soft tissue column found buccally (Kois 1996). This further magnifies the degree of gingival festooning that tends to flatten out towards the posterior sextants of the mouth. Some authors have speculated on the variation in the extent of the biological width and sulcus depth in the different periodontal biotypes (Muller & Eger 2002). Despite the academic interest in these observations it should be remembered that, irrespectively of the degree of scalloping (periodontal biotype), the biological width of a tooth is invariably located supracrestally. The fibers of the connective tissue attachment, functionally inserted into the cementum as Sharpey's fibers, support the gingival margin and the papilla (Fig. 16.10).

In other terms the papilla, supported by the interproximal peaks of bone, can "climb" higher thanks to the additional support that comes from the connective tissue attachment to the tooth.

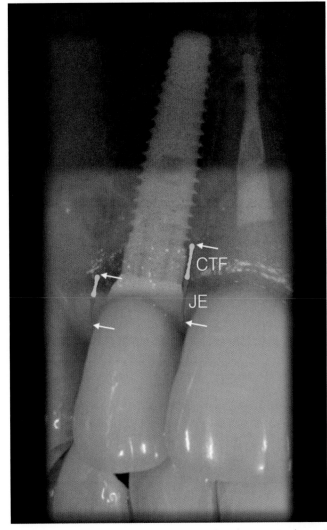

Figure 16.10 The sum of the connective tissue attachment (CTF) and the junctional epithelium (JE) forms the biological width (between the white arrows). A biological width around a tooth forms above the crest of bone differently from how it surrounds an implant, where it forms below the level of the bone.

As previously reported there are several differences between the features of the tooth's biologic dimension and the implant's biologic width, such as their length (about 2 mm for the former and 4 mm for the latter) and their histological and vascular characterization (Glauser et al. 2005). The majority of the information that we have regarding the implant biological seal is derived from animal studies, with only a limited amount of data originating from human experiments.

Similar to what happens in natural dentition, the peri-implant seal has been shown to preserve the homeostasis of the internal environment from external challenges, thus protecting the underlying bone and the developing, or already attained, osseointegration phenomenon (Linkevicius & Apse 2008).

While the different surgical approaches (one-stage, two-stage) (Ericsson et al. 1996) and loading protocols (immediate, early, conventional) do not seem to alter significantly the peri-implant biological dimension (Bakaeen et al. 2009), some human histological evidence reported smaller average values of the tissues surrounding the implant (length of the sulcular epithelium 1.2 ± 0.1 mm, dimension of the junctional epithelium 1.2 ± 0.2 mm, value of the connective tissue fibers 0.6 ± 0.2 mm) for implants designed with a cone-morse connection (Degidi et al. 2012). In light of older information (Hermann et al. 2000) and more recent literature it may be speculated that different implant designs may affect the dimension of the biological seal.

The different microstructure of the implant surfaces adjoining the soft tissues can affect the development of the biological width. It has been shown in human histology how a machined surface favors epithelial downgrowth differently than the rough implant collar, of oxidized or acid-etched implants, where the length of the epithelium was shorter with a longer connective tissue seal (Glauser et al. 2005).

The reported data has shown how the depth of insertion of the implant may affect peri-implant soft tissue dimension (Todescan et al. 2002). The published histomorphometry seems to suggest a trend towards longer junctional epithelium and connective tissue components with deeper implant positioning. In the submerged implant the position of the implant shoulder in relation to the bone crest seems to affect the dimension of the biological seal; in trans-mucosal implants a similar effect has been ascribed to the location of the implant's smooth–rough border (Todescan et al. 2002).

In light of some of the quoted literature it may be suggested that the deeper the implant shoulder position (or the smooth to rough interface) the longer the biological width.

The influence of cone-morse connections rather than flat-to-flat types may further alter the behavior of the surrounding hard and soft tissues. Less osseous resorption has been measured for subcrestally positioned cone-morse implant connections (Weng et al. 2008; Degidi et al. 2011a).

Recent investigations have speculated on positive effects that micro-grooving of the implant collar or the implant abutment may produce on the development of the biological implant seal (Nevins et al. 2008, 2012).

To summarize some of the concepts reported above, while the submerged versus transmucosal approach, or the loading time, do not seem to alter the formation of a biological seal, the implant micro or macro geometry may play a role and amount to differences in the dimensions of the tissues, which may also be related to the diverse implant–abutment connections.

A deeper positioning of the implant is generally associated with a longer biological width, but this may not hold true for all implants.

In recent years immediate implantation at the time of tooth removal has gained popularity and this approach has been reported to result in a longer epithelial interface (Vignoletti et al. 2009). This observation did not vary when testing four different implant systems (De Sanctis et al. 2010).

Knowledge of the peculiar histological and anatomical features of the dento-gingival junction, different from the peri-implant mucosa, becomes fundamental in order to match the patient's expectations. The clinician has to anticipate, before beginning therapy, the potential cosmetic limitations present in certain known clinical scenarios.

AESTHETIC PREDICTABILITY

The tissue that forms around the trans-mucosal portion of the implant, while initially considered similar to the dento-gingival junction (Berglundh et al. 1991), in fact shows a few significant differences that often limit the predictability of achieving ideal soft tissue profiles. This is particularly true in the inter-implant areas, where the presence or absence of the papillae becomes determinant in the final esthetic result (Tarnow et al. 2003).

The recreation of ideal soft tissue profiles (particularly in the papillary areas) around implants is more predictable in areas of single edentulism than in multiple implant sites (Salama et al. 1998; Grunder 2000; Garber et al. 2001; Tarnow et al. 2003) (Figs. 16.11–16.13).

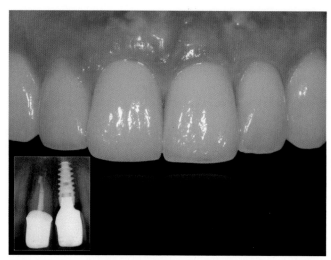

Figure 16.12 Postoperative view. An implant-supported zirconia ceramic crown successfully replaced the left central incisor whereas a zirconia ceramic crown was placed on the right central incisor and a porcelain laminate veneer was cemented on the right lateral incisor. Gingival recontouring was also performed to create better harmony in the final gingival outline. The final periapical X-ray is shown in the lower left corner.

In spite of this, when examining the stability of the buccal mucosal margin around single implants it has been reported how some soft tissue recession has to be expected during the first year following prosthesis insertion (Grunder 2000) (Figs. 16.14 & 16.15). Ten patients were followed for 1 year after single crown insertion and an average 0.6 mm recession was measured. The implants had been placed 8 weeks after

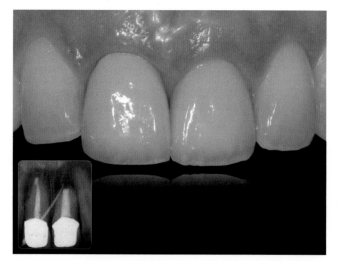

Figure 16.11 Pre-operative view. A single implant is planned to replace the failing left central incisor (note the periapical X-ray in the lower left corner – a gutta-percha cone was inserted into a sinus tract). A guided bone regenerative procedure was necessary prior to implant insertion.

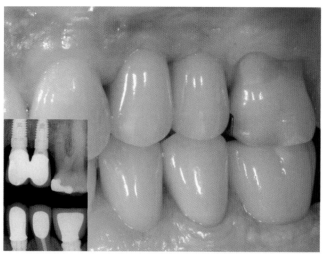

Figure 16.13 Two adjacent implants were placed to restore the two upper left premolars. Note the short and less than ideal papilla in between the two implants. The vertical bitewing X-ray of the area is shown in the lower left corner.

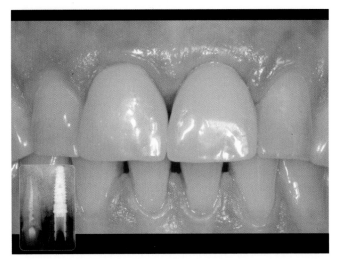

Figure 16.14 The maxillary left central incisor was recently replaced with a temporary implant-supported crown. Note in the clinical picture the proper symmetry of the gingival margins of the central incisors. The X-ray reveals the correct location of the osseous crest to the adjacent teeth but, in spite of this, there is no complete papilla between the centrals.

extraction, with a simultaneous buccal-guided bone regeneration procedure and a connective tissue graft added at the time of membrane removal in the same location (Grunder 2000).

A few years later a 1-year prospective study on 11 single two-stage implants placed in healed edentulous ridges, without any hard or soft tissue augmentation, measured how the facial osseous crest between implant and abutment connection was remodeled (0.7–1.3 mm, $P < 0.05$). No significant changes in the bone could be observed at the interproximal sites. In the

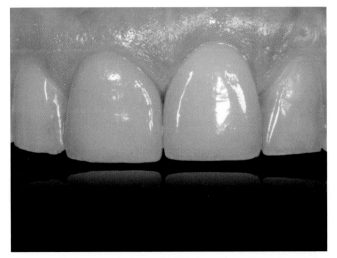

Figure 16.15 Final restoration of implant in Fig. 16.14 after 12 months. Note how the buccal gingival margin has slightly receded on the implant crown while the implant papillae have improved over time.

interval between implant crown insertion and the 12-month follow-up the buccal soft tissue margin receded 0.6 mm while the soft tissue height at proximal sites improved (Cardaropoli et al. 2006).

The apical displacement of the facial mucosal margin around single implants (Chang et al. 1999) was previously reported as an early developing phenomenon in retrospective observations.

A long-term case-control study (minimum 15 years) observed that 27 single-implant crowns were 0.6 ± 1.04 mm longer than the controlateral teeth ($P < 0.05$ mm) at the end of the study (Jemt et al. 2006).

The reported information seems to suggest a tendency for buccal mucosal recession of single-implant restorations. This apical movement of the facial soft tissue has been measured during the first year after crown insertion; during the same period of time, conversely, the single-implant papillae seem to fill the embrasure areas better (Grunder 2000; Cardaropoli et al. 2006; Jemt et al. 2006) (Fig. 16.15).

Similar recessive behavior for the peri-implant tissue margins has been prospectively observed over a 24-month period in 158 multiple implants (Bengazi et al. 1996).

A 1-year prospective study on single and multiple implants confirmed the previous reports, including two-piece and one-piece (transmucosal) implants (Small & Tarnow 2000).

A countertrend observation has been reported by Gallucci et al. in a randomized clinical trial in which stable buccal mucosal margins were measured after crown insertion and over a period of 24 months. The inclusion criteria of the population selected took great care in choosing "ideal" patients for anterior maxillary implants, with presumably voluminous hard and soft tissues that could justify the stable mucosal margins (Gallucci et al. 2011).

Several hypotheses have been formulated to justify this early soft tissue movement. It may be the result of an early remodeling process in order to re-establish proper biological dimensions of the supracrestal soft tissues (the so-called implant biological width of 3–4 mm). This phenomenon may occur because during second-stage surgery an attempt is made to position the tissue margins coronally onto the abutment to create a proper "run way" for the prosthetic components. This unnatural location of the mucosa may progressively recede back to its proper biological distance from the osseous crest (Bengazi et al. 1996).

During peri-implant bone remodeling traditionally about 1 mm of bone is lost during the first year and 0.2 mm per year afterwards (Albrektsson & Zarb 1993), which may affect the final location of the soft tissue margin (Chang et al. 1999).

Multiple connections and disconnections of prosthetic components can disturb the mucosal seal that encircles the implant, causing apical migration of connective tissue and junctional epithelium (Abrahamsson et al. 1997).

To counteract the potentially negative effects of repeated removal of the abutment, clinical strategies have been designed to place the definitive final abutment once, without further manipulation (Rompen et al. 2003; Soadoun & Touati 2007). This "one abutment one time" approach has been investigated with controversial results.

Animal studies have been performed to investigate if multiple disconnections and reconnections of abutments could increase peri-implant bone loss around differently designed implant–abutment complexes. Some authors concluded that the design of the implant–abutment connection could significantly alter the radiographic resorption pattern of the osseous profile and, furthermore, reduce the number of abutment manipulations, which could be useful in reducing bone resorption only for platform-switched implants (see later) but not for matching implant–abutment interfaces (Rodriguez et al. 2013). Unfortunately no undisturbed control group was included in the study by Rodriguez et al. (2013), thus limiting the possible considerations.

Histomorphometrical analysis of animal jaws confirmed the detrimental effect of repeated abutment removal and reconnection on soft and hard tissue levels, and underscored how laser micro-grooved components better preserved bone levels by enhancing subepithelial connective tissue attachment (Iglhaut et al. 2013).

Human prospective clinical trials have been performed in both implant healed sites (Degidi et al. 2011a,b; Grandi et al. 2012) and immediate post-extractive implant sites (Canullo et al. 2010) showing statistically significant reduction of bone loss, when comparing the "one abutment one time" approach with the more traditional approach. In spite of this some researchers (Canullo et al. 2010; Grandi et al. 2012) questioned the clinical relevance of preserving osseous profiles in the order of 0.2–0.3 mm.

A review article published in 2012 concluded that, as well as several other controversial issues regarding features of transmucosal implant components, there is still a severe lack of information regarding the clinical significance of multiple abutment–implant connections on hard and soft tissue remodeling (Rompen 2012).

A short-term (6-month) randomized controlled clinical trial measured a mean marginal bone loss of 0.13 mm for the "one abutment one time" group of implants versus a 0.28 mm osseous resorption for the control group. The difference was found not to be statistically significant and no adverse soft tissue

alterations were caused by the two time abutment disconnection performed in the control group (Koutozis et al. 2013). In spite of the reported results the Koutozis et al. stated in the discussion: "Avoidance of unnecessary disturbance of the transmucosal attachment by multiple abutment disconnections and reconnections is recommended."

Returning to the previous hypothesis on peri-implant soft tissue recession and its relationship with the early remodeling of the implant's osseous profile, clinical considerations, as well as published evidence, ensure this is still a hot topic and open to debate.

A large multi-center prospective clinical study on more than 2500 implants reported how vertical facial osseous resorption at the time of implant uncovering was a common finding when the thickness of the residual bone buccal to the implant osteotomy, at stage I surgery, was less than 1.8 mm. The thinner the residual bone the higher the vertical loss of the buccal osseous crest (Spray et al. 2000).

The tridimensional shape of the osseous "saucerization" that traditionally forms around the implant neck has been the focus of clinical considerations when placing implants in the esthetic zone (Grunder et al. 2005). A minimum of 2 mm of bone buccal to the implant has been advocated to avoid the risk of losing bone height and thus increasing the possibility of soft tissue recession (Buser et al. 2004).

To avoid the potential esthetic detrimental effect resulting from the spatial relationship between the location of the implant platform and the often too thin osseous plate facial to it, several clinical and technological solutions have been proposed. A common clinical strategy that has been reported to be successful is to horizontally thicken the facial bone through guided bone regeneration irrespective of the presence, or not, of an osseous dehiscence or fenestration buccal to the implant (Grunder et al. 2005; Cosyn & De Rouck 2009) (Figs. 16.16–16.18).

In the paper published by Cosyn & De Rouck in 2009 it is interesting to note how there was no apical recession of the facial mucosal margin, which is different from what was previously noted by Grunder in 2000.

It is possible that this non-negligible difference when discussing esthetic predictability could be ascribed to the use of a resorbable barrier by the latter group instead of the previously reported e-PTFE material. The use of an absorbable material allowed the Belgian group to use a significantly more conservative surgical approach on the treated patients (fewer surgeries and less invasive).

To further confirm the positive esthetic results obtained with this surgical approach, two prospective studies with follow-ups at

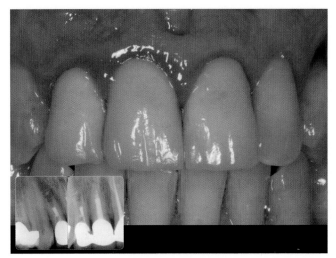

Figure 16.16 A single implant is planned to replace the failing maxillary right lateral incisor.

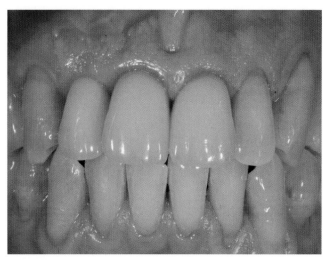

Figure 16.18 Follow-up of the final restoration of the implant shown in Figs. 16.16 and 16.17.

12 and 36 months have been published. The authors reported a 5% incidence (1 case out of 20 followed) of limited facial mucosal recession (between 0.5 and 1 mm), revealing generally pleasing esthetic outcomes for the population undergoing the research (Buser et al. 2009, 2011).

Regarding the several technological advancements now offered by many implant producers to improve the performance of the devices in terms of bone response, some of the reported literature should be examined in depth (Weng et al. 2008; Nevins et al. 2008, 2012; Iglhaut et al. 2013; Degidi et al. 2011, 2012; Rodriguez et al. 2013).The quest for the ideal implant design in terms of bone response and osseous preservation is still ongoing and needs to be further investigated.

It is also worth mentioning at this point how depending on the peri-implant mucosal biotype marginal bone loss might not influence or impair the esthetic result.

Retrospective sketchy observations from the mid-1990s came to the conclusion that exposed implant threads do not necessarily lead to subsequent mucosal problems (Lekholm et al. 1996).

A recent narrative review concluded that there is not sufficient evidence linking bone level to future mucosal recession (Cairo et al. 2008).

A systematic review failed to correlate the facial bone dimension with the esthetic results of therapy and a minimal buccal bone

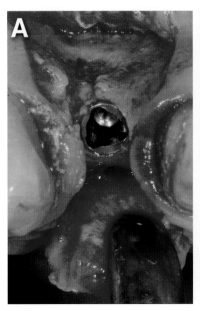
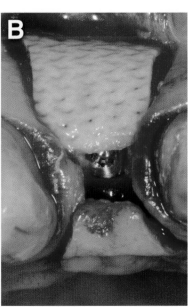

Figure 16.17 (A) During implant placement the buccal cortical bone appears thinner than 2 mm. (B) A resorbable membrane is placed on top of a bone graft to thicken the osseous anatomy.

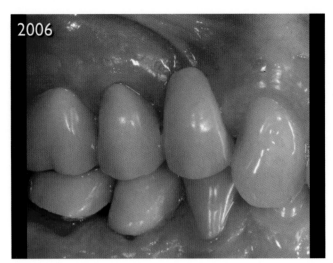

2006

Figure 16.19 Pre-operative view of the edentulous area of the first maxillary bicuspid. Note the marked concavity of the area and the frenum insertion.

thickness threshold, critical to optimal esthetic, could not be set for the paucity of relevant bibliographical information available (Teughels et al. 2009).

A radiological cross-sectional retrospective evaluation of a pool of patients was performed on 14 immediate implants subjected to simultaneous guided bone regeneration. At a 7-year follow-up the clinically re-examined patients underwent a cone beam exam that revealed how 5 implants out of 14 (35.7%) were missing the buccal bone. In spite of a major difference in the location of the facial implant crest level between those with or without the buccal bone, the difference in the position of the mucosal margin amounted to as little as 1 mm (Benic et al. 2012).

By gathering all the previous observations it could be speculated that apical movement in the buccal crest of bone may not be followed by similar recession of the mucosal margin when the soft tissue resists thanks to its thickness. It has been reported in a retrospective cross-sectional study on single anterior implants that a thin biotype appears to be the most relevant factor in determining the facial marginal mucosal level, with a statistically significant odds ratio of 18.8 (Nisapakultorn et al. 2010).

The presence of a well-represented and stable osseous scaffold underneath the facial mucosal margin grants a certain stability and resistance to it and procedures that augment the bone in the esthetic area should probably be routinely employed to this end.

At the same time thickening the buccal peri-implant soft tissue, particularly in the presence of a thin biotype, is advisable and makes it more resistant to recession even in the presence of unfavorable osseous defects (Schneider et al. 2011) (Figs. 16.19–16.23).

A publication on single implants in the esthetic zone stressed the difference between the length of interproximal soft tissue on the implant side (4–6.5 mm/implant platform, top of the papilla) and the same distance on the adjacent tooth side (3–4.5 mm/interproximal osseous peak, top of the papilla) (Smukler et al. 2003). It is now widely accepted that under such clinical circumstances the height of the papilla is maintained by the interproximal osseous crest on the adjacent natural tooth (Salama et al. 1998; Grunder 2000; Smukler et al. 2003a,b)

The presence of a thick and flat biotype increases the predictability of a pleasant esthetic result. Thick tissues are in fact

Figure 16.20 Occlusal view of the edentulous area of the case depicted in Fig. 16.19. (A) Preoperative view. (B) Same view of the area after implant placement with concomitant guided bone regeneration used to thicken the buccal osseous structure. Note the significant change in the buccal soft tissue profile.

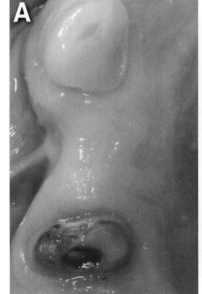
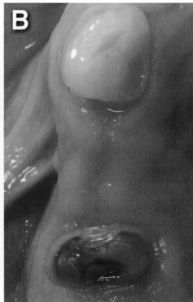

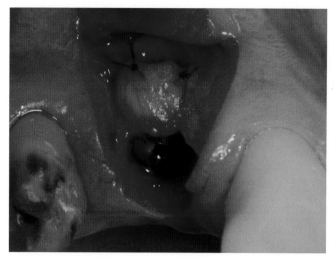

Figure 16.21 During second-stage surgery a peduncolated soft tissue graft is obtained by flipping buccally the connective tissue plug that was lying on top of the cover screw.

more resistant to the controlled traumatic injuries caused during dental treatments, while a lower degree of scalloping in the gingiva is more easily replicable at the end of implant therapy. For obvious reasons it is easier to replace a missing tooth in a periodontally treated patient and obtain soft tissue profiles that are in harmony with the remaining natural dentition (Figs. 16.24–16.26) A human retrospective study evaluated the dimensions of the peri-implant mucosa of 45 maxillary single implants in the aesthetic zone (Kan et al. 2003). The measurements of the peri-implant mucosa performed at the mesial, mid-facial, and distal locations were obtained with a periodontal probe inserted under local anesthesia until contact was made with the osseous crest (bone sounding). A comparison was made between the data procured in the thick versus thin periodontal biotypes, and the authors concluded that "at all evaluated

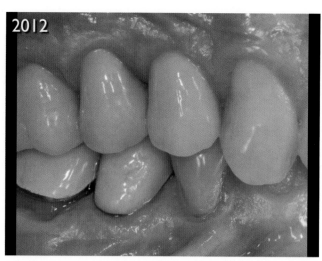

Figure 16.23 Four-year follow-up of the final crown on the implant shown in Figs. 16.19–16.22 after guided bone regeneration and connective tissue thickening of the area. Note the major improvement in the quantity and quality of the tissue surrounding the implant.

sites, greater peri-implant mucosal dimensions were noted in the presence of the thick periodontal biotype" even if statistical significance was reached only for the mesial location.

In the natural dentition with a distance of 5 mm or less from the contact point to the osseous crest the papilla was reported to completely fill the embrasure space in 98% of cases (Tarnow et al. 1992). A similar observation performed for single implants (Choquet et al. 2001) measured the presence of an almost ideal papilla in 88% of cases when the distance between the contact point and the crest of bone adjacent to the natural tooth

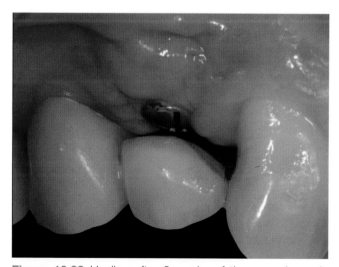

Figure 16.22 Healing after 2 weeks of the area shown in Fig. 16.21.

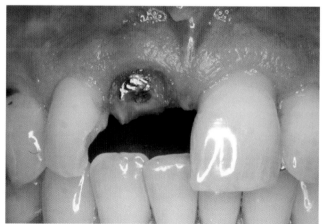

Figure 16.24 Pre-operative view. The right central incisor is fractured and scheduled for extraction and immediate implant placement. The crown of the right lateral incisor is fractured as well, and a composite resin restoration will be done. Note the flat and thick biotype and the marginal recession of the gingival tissues.

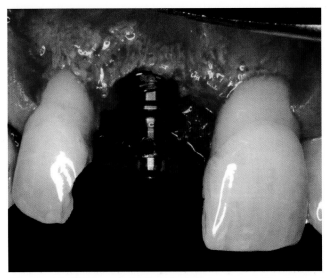

Figure 16.25 Immediate implant placement at the time of extraction.

was 5 mm or less. While similar behavior was reported in the interdental area and the embrasure space between an implant and a natural tooth, it should be noticed that a slight difference (12%) in the percentage of papillae existed in the two different clinical scenarios.

To obtain an almost 100% presence of papillae entirely filling the embrasures between a dental element and an implant the reported measured distance was 3 mm or less.

The possibility of predictably recreating an ideal gingival outline between two or more contiguous implants has been questioned (Tarnow et al. 2003) (Fig. 16.13). Whenever the rehabilitation involves two or more lost teeth, the osseous profile of the edentulous area (matched by the gingival profile) is no

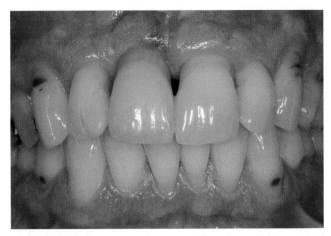

Figure 16.26 Seven-year follow-up. Despite a slight marginal disharmony between the two centrals, the overall esthetic result is acceptable because of the generalized gingival recession pattern and the flat biotype of the patient.

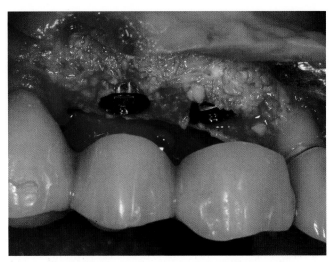

Figure 16.27 Two implants are placed after healing of a guided bone regeneration procedure that was previously performed to straighten the concave osseous anatomy of the area. Note the proper spacing of the implants, which should encourage maintenance of the inter-implant osseous crest height.

longer scalloped but either flat or, worse, concave. This means no longer having that precious interproximal osseous septum that normally supports the papilla. It is nowadays possible, and advisable, to transform a concave edentulous ridge into a flat one through the use of guided bone regeneration (GBR) procedures (Jovanovic & Nevins 1995; Simion et al. 1994). In the best case scenario starts with a flat osseous anatomy into which the implants will be inserted (Fig. 16.27). According to some authors, with proper mesio-distal spacing of the fixtures (more than 3 mm) a better maintenance of the inter-implant bone height is obtained (Tarnow et al. 2000) (Fig. 16.28). In a human retrospective report from Tarnow et al., the average loss of height of the osseous septum between the fixtures is 1.04 mm for implants placed up to 3 mm apart; when the implants were more than 3 mm apart the vertical loss of bone was 0.45 mm. A later experiment conducted on dogs seems to confirm the different behavior of inter-implant bone depending on the distance between adjacent implants (Scarano et al. 2004). The vertical loss of crestal bone between implants decreased from 1.98 mm when implants were spaced 2 mm from each other, to 0.23 mm with a spacing distance of 5 mm.

The distance between contiguous implants immediately placed and restored, and its influence on the aesthetic result, was evaluated in a human retrospective observation by Degidi et al. (2008). At 1 year from insertion of the final restoration a better aesthetic result was achieved for adjacent implants placed at a distance of more than 2 mm and less than 4 mm. It is interesting to notice how on an average the implants used in Tarnow's research experienced a loss of bone, lateral to the implant platform, of around 1.4 mm versus an average value of

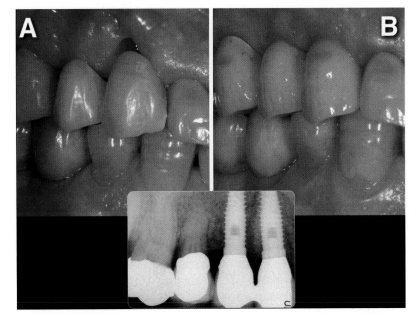

Figure 16.28 (A) Pre-operative view of the area implanted in Fig. 16.27. Note the significant soft tissue defect present in the canine area. (B) Completed case; a harmonious soft tissue profile has been recreated. In the lower part of the picture the 1-year follow-up X-ray displays a stable inter-implant osseous crest. Some deproteinized bovine bone used during hard tissue augmentation is still detectable.

about 0.6 mm for the implants utilized by Degidi et al. The different macro and micro geometry of the implants used probably explains the different osseous responses.

More recent animal research (Arthur et al. 2006) performed with morse cone and platform-switched connection implants did not confirm the previous human retrospective observations (Tarnow et al. 2000) or animal experiments (Scarano et al. 2004). No significant difference was found in terms of peri-implant bone response when the implants were spaced at 1, 2, or 3 mm; under every experimental condition bone resorbed in a similar manner, irrespectively of the inter-implant distance. The different conclusions between studies can be explained by the diverse designs of the investigations and, in particular, the difficulties encountered in trying to reproduce the human alveolar ridge in animal models.

It also possible, once again, that the dissimilar implant designs utilized by the authors influenced different osseous behaviors. Confirmation of this can be found in the article by Weng et al. (2008) in which the authors came to the conclusion that: "different microgap designs cause different shapes and sizes of the peri-implant ('dish-shaped') bone defect in submerged implants both in equicrestal and subcrestal positions".

A later publication by the same Brazilian group (Arthur et al. 2009) on a similar animal model and with an immediate loading approach came to similar conclusions. No significant differences, in terms of crestal resorption or inter-implant papillae formation, were measured between implants spaced at 2 or 3 mm apart. What appeared to be significant for the implant design utilized (morse cone and platform-switched connection implants) was the subcrestal implant placement, which, compared to a crestal placement, had a positive impact on papillae

formation and osseous remodeling with bone located slightly above the top of the implants. The same group later reported the histomorphometrical measurements of the aforementioned animals, with results in accordance with the previous conclusions (Barros et al. 2010).

The inter-implant peak of bone, when present, is often located more apical than the one that existed before the loss of the natural dental elements. Additionally, the two contiguous implants do not possess Sharpey's fibers functionally inserted into the cementum to support the supracrestal soft tissue (Tarnow et al. 2003). The biological width around two-stage implants ad modum Brånemark always forms subcrestally (Berglundh and Lindhe 1996). In this process bone is resorbed (360° around the neck of the implant) and replaced by connective tissue fibers. Whether this is the result of the biological width forming (Berglundh & Lindhe 1996) or due to the cupping phenomenon caused by the bacterial contamination of the microgap (Hermann et al. 1997, 2000), the final result does not change. The connective tissue encircling the fixtures starts subcrestally differently from what happens around natural teeth where the supracrestal connective tissue fibers further support the verticality of the gingival tissue (Tarnow et al. 2003).

When one considers that, according to the data we have available (Tarnow et al. 2003), the average height of the inter-implant soft tissue (measured from the inter-implant peak of bone to the tip of the papilla) is equal to 3.4 mm, it is easy to understand the esthetic limitations that we encounter when placing two adjacent implants in the cosmetic zone.

This value of about 3.5 mm has been somewhat confirmed by others (Arthur et al. 2006) who report a measurement of 3,7 mm.

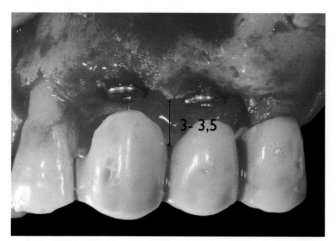

Figure 16.29 Intraoperative view of adjacent implants. Note the proper spacing between the two fixtures and the provisional in place to anticipate the 3–3.5 mm distance between the osseous crest and the prosthetic contact point.

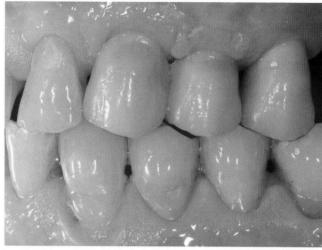

Figure 16.31 Final prosthetic restoration of case depicted in Fig. 16.29. In order to avoid a black triangle the contact point was lowered to a distance of 3 mm from the osseous crest.

Following what was just reported, in an attempt to obtain a complete closure of the embrasure space between adjacent implants, Degidi et al. (2008) suggested a 3–4 mm distance between the contact point and the inter-implant osseous peak. A human retrospective study evaluated the effect of the same vertical distance on the presence of an inter-proximal papilla and suggested 3 mm for adjacent implants (Gastaldo et al. 2004). Similar advice can be found in a review paper (Chow & Wang 2010) in which, between the conditions favoring the inter-implant papilla appearance, a 3 mm distance between the restorations contact point and the crest of bone was advocated.

The 2004 retrospective observation by Gastaldo et al. (2004) examined the effect of the vertical distance from the contact point to the crest of bone and the horizontal spacing between an implant and a tooth or a second implant on the incidence of an ideal interproximal papilla that completely filled the embrasure space.

An ideal papilla was present in the embrasure between adjacent implants when the vertical distance contact point-crest of inter-implant bone was equal to 3 mm; the same ideal papilla was found between an implant and a natural dental element for vertical distances of 3 and 4 mm. The lateral spacing between two implants or an implant and a tooth that allowed for the creation of an ideal papilla was reported to be 3–4 mm (Figs. 16.29–16.31). The authors also suggest that other factors may play a role in the papilla formation, such as the bucco-lingual

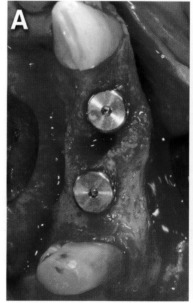
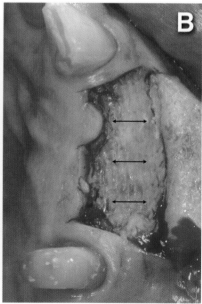

Figure 16.30 (A) Intraoperative occlusal view of the two implants of Fig. 16.29 before guided bone regeneration. (B) After guided bone regeneration the implants are submerged into newly formed osseous tissue. Note the significant thickening (black arrows) of the bone buccal to the implants.

dimension of the inter-proximal osseous septum. The same idea is suggested in the publication by Grunder et al. (2005) in which they found that horizontal thickening of the interproximal bone peak through GBR may improve the presence and stability of the papilla (Fig. 16.30). Retrospective research performed to evaluate the effects of bucco-palatal bone width on the incidence of inter-proximal papilla between implants could not confirm these hypotheses (Siqueira et al. 2013). In spite of the lack of statistical significance that the authors report relative to the influence of bucco-palatal width of bone and presence of inter-implant papilla, when the width of the crest was less than 4 mm the papilla was always absent while it was present in 36.4% of the cases for dimensions of 4 mm or more. In the discussion it is mentioned how the statistics may well be affected by the lack of power of the small sample size and it is concluded that further studies with more participants are required to fully investigate the matter.

ONE-PIECE IMPLANTS VS TWO-PIECE IMPLANTS

Investigations on one-piece non-submerged implants (ITI implants; Straumann, Basel, Switzerland) have shown different patterns in the way crestal bone heals around the fixture when compared to two-piece implants (Hermann et al. 2001) (Figs. 16.32–16.35).

According to Hermann et al., in a flat-to-flat connection two-piece implant the presence of a microgap in the vicinity of the osseous crest determines the increased resorption of bone when compared to a one-stage one-piece implant.

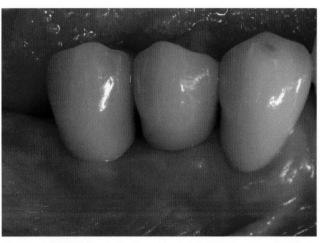

Figure 16.33 After reflection of a full-thickness flap, the deficient buccolingual width of the edentulous ridge is obvious.

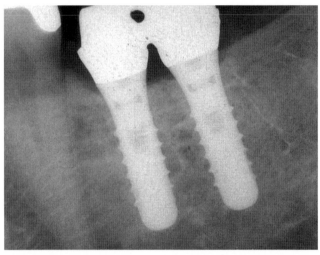

Figure 16.34 Radiograph showing the peri-implant osseous resorption pattern around one-piece transmucosal implants. Note the different resorption pattern from the two-stage submerged type of implants (compare with Fig. 16.32).

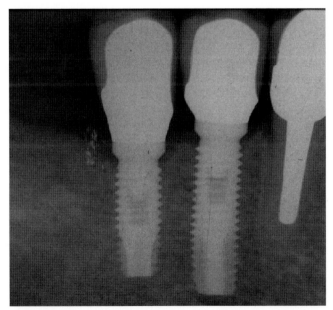

Figure 16.32 Pre-operative view of the area planned for an implant-supported restoration. There is a lack of proper bone width in the edentulous area.

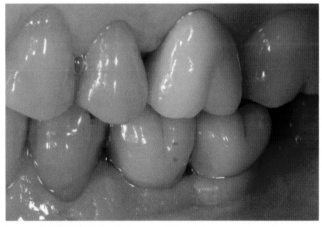

Figure 16.35 Clinical picture of the two one-piece transmucosal implants shown in Fig. 16.34.

In the 1990s animal investigations conducted in Sweden showed that multiple disconnections and reconnections of the implant abutment were followed by a more apical relocation of the peri-implant connective tissue band (Abrahamsson et al. 1997). It seems reasonable to assume that a transmucosal implant design, which presents with a prosthetic interface located away from the osseous crest and in a iuxta-gingival position, would better respect the integrity both of the osseous tissue and the soft tissues encircling the fixture.

The average biological width dimension measured for a one-piece implant (2.84 mm) is similar to the one found around a natural tooth (2.73 mm = biologic width + sulcus depth) and is generally smaller than the one measured around a two-piece implant (Ericsson et al. 1996; Hermann et al. 2001). The Brånemark type of implant is additionally characterized by a more apical location of the gingival margin when compared to an ITI type of fixture (Hermann et al. 2001).

As well as the evidence presented by Hermann et al. (2001), conducted on a dog model, one-piece, one-stage implants were also included in the investigation conducted by Tarnow et al. on 136 interimplant papillae measuring on an average of 3.4 mm (Tarnow et al. 2003). The recessive behavior measured within the first year for single and multiple implants was also present in the transmucosal implant design (Small & Tarnow 2000).

According to the value reported by Kois (1996) the average papillary height in the natural dentition is usually around 4.5 mm, about 1 mm more than what was measured between implants. Furthermore, the interimplant peak of bone, in spite of advancements obtained with osseous regenerative procedures, is commonly found to be more apical than the original interdental osseous crest. This is particularly true in the presence of a scalloped periodontal biotype.

To improve the esthetic result in the cosmetic zone, the ITI type of fixture is commonly sunk more apically to produce a transmucosal space. This space is used to develop an ideal anatomic profile with prosthetic components that connect to the otherwise un-anatomical round platform of the implant. In doing this the rough–smooth interface of the implant is buried deeper in the bone and, according to Hermann et al. (1997, 2000), this determines a larger circumferential loss of crestal bone. Under this circumstance the differences between one-stage and two-stage implants are minimal, if they exist at all.

In the attempt to overcome these limitations new scalloped fixture designs have been proposed (Holt et al. 2002) and introduced into the market (Wöhrle 2003). A 1-year randomized clinical trial comparing hard and soft tissue changes on 20 patients treated with a scalloped fixture design versus 20 patients treated with a flat implant design reported worse bone

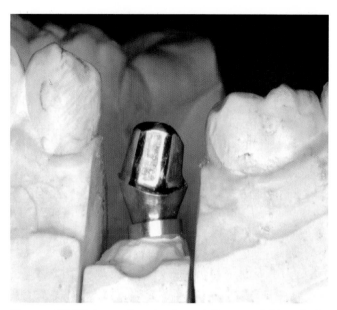

Figure 16.36 According to the platform-switching technique, a 4-mm diameter abutment is used on a 5-mm diameter implant platform. Here an anatomical custom abutment has been manufactured.

loss around the scalloped implants and no difference in the papilla index or patient satisfaction (Tymstra et al. 2011).

With the knowledge that crestal bone remodels away, both vertically and horizontally, from the implant–abutment interface (Tarnow et al. 2000), several clinicians have successfully managed to minimize the peri-implant osseous "cupping" by moving the microgap inward. This clinical intuition, called the platform-switching technique, can be easily accomplished (with certain implant types) by reducing the diameter of the abutment (e.g., 4 mm abutment platform) in relation to the supporting implant diameter (e.g., 5 mm implant platform) (Figs. 16.36–16.38).

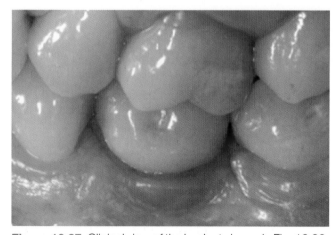

Figure 16.37 Clinical view of the implant shown in Fig. 16.36.

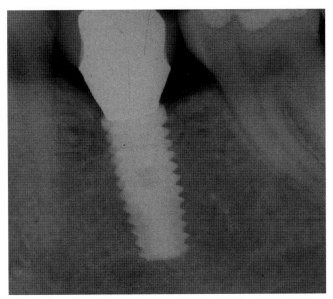

Figure 16.38 Radiograph of the implant depicted in Fig. 16.27. Note how the platform-switching approach seems to abate the amount of peri-implant bone loss.

It is relevant to note how some implant manufacturers have in the past designed their fixtures with a coronal bevel that brings the abutment to sit inside the implant platform. Research comparing this design (Astra Tech implants) to the more traditional Brånemark fixture produced controversial results regarding differences in the amount of crestal bone resorption. Independently from the significance or not of the compared average value of the vertical osseous loss around the two systems, there was common agreement on the different initial pattern of bone remodeling noted for the beveled platform (Puchades-Roman et al. 2000; Astrand et al. 2004).

Nowadays more implant companies have shaped their implants with a built-in platform-switched/shifted connection in an attempt to ameliorate peri-implant crestal osseous resorption (Fig. 16.39). A randomized controlled trial, performed over a period of almost 3 years on 80 implants in 31 patients, came to the conclusion that marginal bone levels were better maintained in implants restored with the platform-switching concept (Canullo et al. 2010). The same research also measured an inverse correlation between the extent of mismatch and the amount of bone loss.

To further validate the concept a systematic review was published in 2010, comprising 10 studies including 1239 implants, and reported a significant decrease in marginal bone loss (mean difference of −0.37 mm, 95% CI: −0.55 to −0.20, $P < 0.0001$) for platform-switched implants (Atieh et al. 2010).

A subgroup analysis highlighted how a mismatch of ≥0.4 mm was associated with a more favorable bone response.

UNCOVERING TECHNIQUES

When a submerged approach is selected a second surgery is performed for several purposes: it allows the implant to be uncovered and the achievement of clinical osseointegration verified, it permits the connection of the healing abutment or the provisional restoration with the fixture, and last but not least it represents the last chance to improve the peri-implant soft tissue. At the second stage of surgery the clinician should carefully

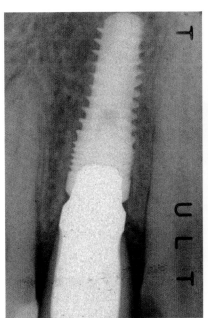

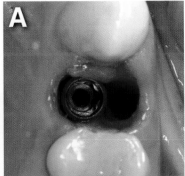

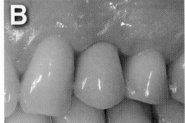

Figure 16.39 (A) A built-in platform-switched design characterizes the implant selected to be immediately placed in the first bicuspid socket. (B) Final implant-supported crown in place. The peri-apical X-ray on the left shows excellent marginal osseous profiles with bone persisting, coronal to the implant platform, in close proximity to the implant prosthetic components.

evaluate the site to determine if the quantity and quality of the soft tissues fulfills the previously planned therapy expectations.

Unfortunately, more often than what we would desire, deficits in terms of volume of tissue or keratinization of the gingiva (or both) will be present. Whenever possible an adequate peri-implant keratinized tissue (2 mm at least) should be obtained from adjacent sites through the use of pedicle flaps (Moy et al. 1989; Hertel et al. 1994). If the surrounding anatomy does not favor the sculpting of a pedicle flap, the alternative naturally falls on epithelialized soft tissue grafts (Sullivan & Atkins 1968). If the amount of keratinized tissue present in the area is reduced but not completely absent (approximately 1 mm), it is possible nowadays to consider the use of xenografts to increase the keratinization of the peri-implant mucosa (Sanz et al. 2009).

For bucco-lingual volumetric defects, modifications of the original Abrams's roll technique can be successfully utilized (Abrams 1980; Scharf & Tarnow 1992; Israelson & Plemons 1993; Barone et al. 1999). The peri-implant soft tissue can also be augmented by grafting connective tissue either before or at the time of the uncovering (Langer & Calagna 1980; Silverstein et al. 1994; Hurzeler & Weng 1996).

In the attempt to recreate the lost papillary tissues between implants several techniques have been proposed (Salama et al. 1995; Adriaenssens et al. 1999; Palacci & Ericsson 2001; Tinti & Benfenati 2002; Smukler et al. 2003a). In spite of the good clinical intuitions of the authors, the predictability of the different approaches is yet to be scientifically proven.

Other reports have addressed the surgical removal of a non-resorbable membrane during second-stage surgery (Landi & Sabatucci 2001).

The ever-increasing need for guided bone regeneration of implant recipient sites (Grunder et al. 2005) justifies the interest in new uncovering techniques. While the expanding use of resorbable membranes has mitigated the problems related to barrier removal (Zitzmann et al. 1997; Friedmann et al. 2002), other drawbacks consequential to previous regenerative procedures still deserve some consideration.

The necessity for primary wound closure over a membrane, independently from its biodegradable properties, often results in a coronal displacement of the muco-gingival tissues. In many cases this further reduces the already deficient amount of gingiva that overlies the edentulous ridge and surrounds the adjacent teeth.

Flap designs that aim at minimizing the coronal displacement of the muco-gingival junction at the time of membrane placement should be utilized whenever possible (Tinti & Parma-Benfenati 1995; Nemcovsky et al. 1999, 2000; Triaca et al. 2001). If the anatomy of the treated area does not permit the use of such

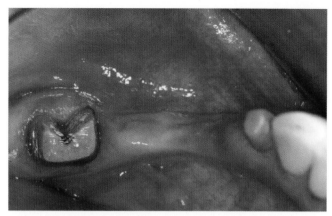

Figure 16.40 Pre-operative view of the area planned for an implant-supported restoration. There is a lack of proper bone width in the edentulous area.

techniques the second-stage surgery should be planned to compensate for the lost muco-gingival relationship (Rosenquist 1997). This means utilizing well-known periodontal plastic procedures (repositioned pedicle flaps, free gingival grafts, connective tissue grafts, etc.) to regain the proper lost anatomical landmarks (Figs. 16.40–6.52).

Tissue-Punch Uncovering Technique

This approach has its origin in the original description of second-stage surgery by P.-I. Brånemark (Adell et al. 1981). The technique was originally devised for implant-supported restorations of fully edentulous patients and did not give any consideration to the final esthetic outcome of the peri-implant soft tissues.

To quote the words of Rosenquist (1997) regarding the esthetics of the gingival tissues abut an implant: "four factors are important: 1) the width and position of the attached gingiva; 2) the buccal volume of the alveolar process; 3) the level and

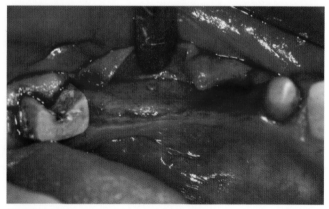

Figure 16.41 After reflection of a full-thickness flap, the deficient buccolingual width of the edentulous ridge is obvious.

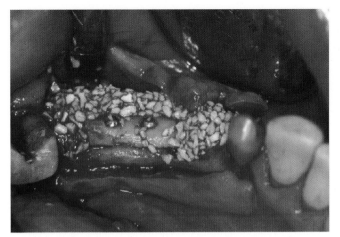

Figure 16.42 A block graft taken from the mandibular ramus, immediately posterior to the area, is secured in place with two fixation screws. An additional particulate xenograft is used to fill the voids and increase the volume of the graft.

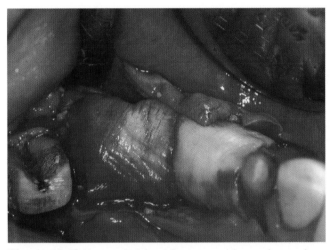

Figure 16.43 A resorbable collagen membrane is used on top of the graft.

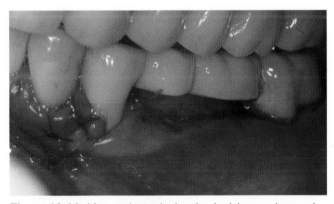

Figure 16.44 After periosteal releasing incisions, primary closure of the wound is achieved. In this maneuver, the mucogingival line is displaced coronally. Note how the provisional restoration has been adjusted to compensate for swelling in the area.

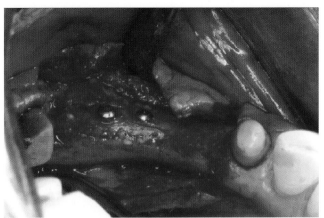

Figure 16.45 After 6 months of healing, the area is reopened. There is excellent graft integration and successful osseous regeneration.

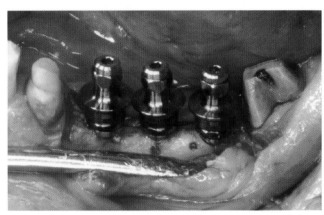

Figure 16.46 Three standard-diameter implants are placed.

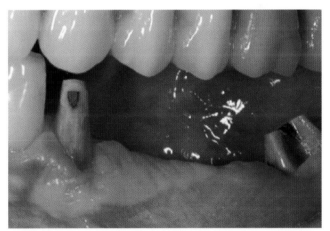

Figure 16.47 The day of the uncovering. The coronal displacement of the mucogingival line, in the edentulous space immediately mesial to the residual second molar, is still noticeable.

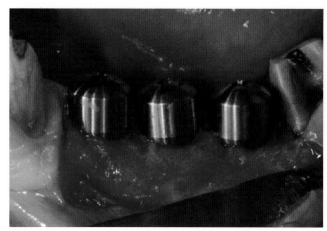

Figure 16.48 A partial-thickness flap is reflected and the temporary healing abutments are placed.

configuration of the gingival margin; and 4) the size and shape of the papillae."

This approach presents the unique advantage of exposing only the head of the implant, thus minimizing the surgical trauma, and is indicated only in ideal circumstances. In other words, any time the four conditions mentioned above are satisfied before the uncovering of the fixture, it becomes advisable to use this technique.

In any other case the use of a tissue-punch approach would further reduce an already deficient width of keratinized gingiva and make it impossible to correct for soft tissue discrepancies.

A few more drawbacks that have to be mentioned are that with the tissue-punch approach there is no visibility of the implant/bone interface and moreover, due to the bleeding, it

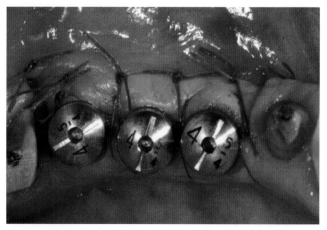

Figure 16.49 The flap is buccally and apically repositioned with 5-0 vicryl external mattress sutures. Single interrupted sutures are used to close the two vertical-releasing incisions. The mucogingival line has been newly moved toward its original, more apical, position.

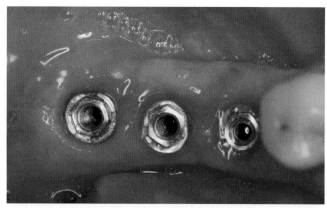

Figure 16.50 After healing of the area, the width of the ridge appears significantly increased as a result of the osseous augmentation (compare with Fig. 16.40). The uncovering technique provided the fixtures with an adequate amount of keratinized mucosa surrounding them. By 4 weeks after the second-stage surgery, there is good healing of the area.

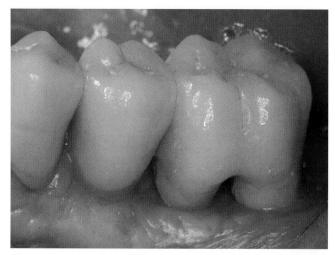

Figure 16.51 Final restoration in place.

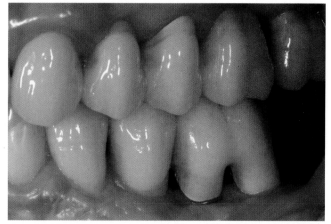

Figure 16.52 Six-year follow-up of the case shown in Fig. 16.51. A slight recession of the peri-implant mucosal margin is noticeable on the middle implant. Mucosal tissues are otherwise stable and healthy.

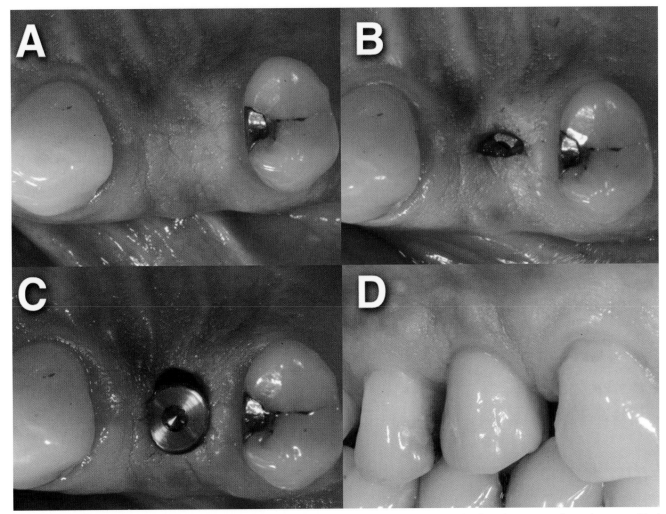

Figure 16.53 (A) An ideal quality and quantity of the tissues in the previously implanted edentulous area allows for a modified tissue punch technique. (B) The initial half-moon incision is designed palatally with a blade no. 15C to find and expose the palatal half of the fixture head. (C) Completion of the modified tissue punch incision is performed towards the buccal side. (D) Final implant-supported crown in place. Note the good quality and quantity of the peri-implant mucosal tissues.

can be more difficult to evaluate the proper seating of the abutment. Peri-implant osseous resorptions that developed during the healing after first-stage surgery can go undiagnosed, and it becomes mandatory to take an X-ray to verify the correct seating of the abutment.

This procedure, which does not require any suturing, results in minimal postoperative discomfort for the patient, who can start brushing the area right away, and can be easily accomplished with a dedicated punch-blade or blade no. 15C (modified tissue-punch technique) (Fig. 16.53).

Apically Positioned Flap

The transposition of periodontal surgical techniques to implant-uncovering procedures was a natural evolution in the emerging field of implant therapy (Moy et al. 1989).

As previously mentioned, the presence of keratinized tissue surrounding implants, although not fundamental for the survival of the fixture, is supported by biological (Nevins & Mellonig 1998), functional (Alpert 1994), and esthetic reasons (Saadoun & LeGall 1992).

The significance of the depth of the peri-implant sulcus has been the object of many investigations. From the initial clinical research that minimized the clinical significance of the peri-implant probing depth (Apse et al. 1991), developed the awareness of its importance in order to prevent and avoid biological complications (Lang et al. 2000). It has been shown that a shallow peri-implant sulcus corresponds to a microbial flora distinctive of soft tissue health and vice versa (Dharmar et al. 1994).

On the basis of these considerations, the establishment of a firm band of keratinized tissue surrounding a fixture, which

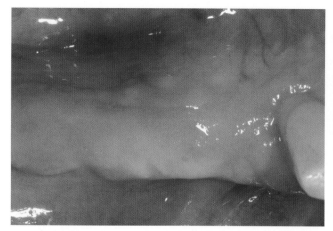

Figure 16.54 Pre-operative view. Three implants are buried under the tissue. Note the position of the mucogingival line. An apical repositioning of the keratinized mucosa is advisable to idealize the quality of the tissue surrounding the implants.

presents with a reduced depth of the peri-implant sulcus, is regarded as ideal. The surgical apical repositioning of the gingiva at the time of second-stage surgery is intended to create this ideal scenario.

The biological price of this more invasive approach is counterbalanced by its several advantages: it provides better access to the implant site, allowing the correct seating of the abutment to be confirmed, the soft tissues can be properly thinned, reducing future probing depth, and finally it becomes possible to preserve or even augment the keratinized tissue.

When thinning of the mucosa is deemed necessary to idealize the future depth of the peri-implant sulcus, a flap thickness greater than 2 mm should be preserved. This should

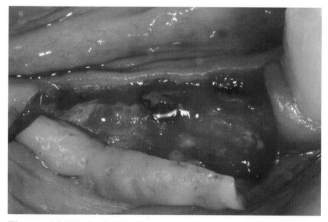

Figure 16.55 A slightly lingual horizontal incision has been designed on the crest, sparing the papilla distal to the canine. Two vertical-releasing incisions have been placed, mesial and distal to the first incision, and a partial-thickness flap has been raised.

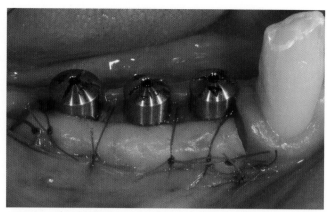

Figure 16.56 After positioning of the healing abutments the flap is sutured apical to its original location.

avoid osseous resorption during healing and accommodate the proper biological width (Berglundh & Lindhe 1996).

The surgical technique is relatively easy to accomplish, although it is more demanding than the punch approach. The author favors the use of a blade no. 15C to sculpt a rectangular, or vaguely trapezoidal, partial thickness flap that exposes the implant platform onto which the abutment is then placed, and is finally sutured apically to the implant's head (Figs. 16.54–16.57).

The use of a partial thickness flap (Fig. 16.55) minimizes the insult to the underlying, often thin, peri-implant osseous anatomy (Staffileno et al. 1966) and allows for an easier control of flap repositioning thanks to periosteal suturing (Fig. 16.56).

For single implants the two vertical releasing incisions are usually kept slightly divergent towards the buccal vestibule to allow better blood supply to the narrower coronal portion of the partial thickness flap (Mormann & Ciancio 1977). The vertical incisions are beveled to improve the healing, reduce the scarring and ease the adaptation of the flap onto its underlying vascular bed (Kon et al. 1984). The inclusion of the papillae in the flap should be avoided whenever the mesio-distal space of the edentulous area is more than 6 mm (Saadoun 1997). While including the papillary areas in the flap would not impair the final formation of nice papillae, if the osseous septum is properly located (Smukler et al. 2003a) the exclusion of them from the flap design allows an immediately mature interproximal tissue to be readily molded by the provisional restoration (Tarnow et al. 2003).

When the mesio-distal space is too constricted (6 mm) it becomes difficult to properly design a flap that spares the papillae, and the coronal portion of the flap would be extremely narrow, with a high risk of necrosis. When the technique is used to uncover multiple implants the two vertical releasing incisions are kept parallel to each other and beveled, as already described. This simplifies the apical sliding of this more

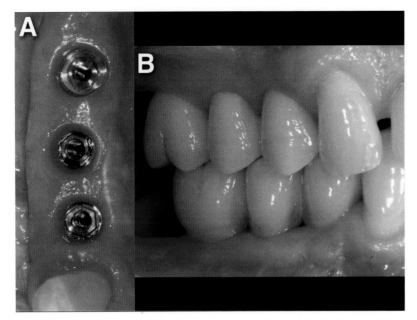

Figure 16.57 (A) Healing of the peri-implant mucosa. Note the ideal keratinized tissue surrounding the implants and the shallow peri-implant sulcus that resulted from the uncovering procedure. (B) Final restoration in place. A good amount of keratinized mucosa is visible buccal to the implants.

rectangular flap in comparison with the previously described trapezoidal flap. For second-stage surgery (of two or more implants) the broader extent of the flap crossed by numerous blood vessels, which give it the correct nutrition, is such that there is no need to widen its base to enrich the blood flow. It is usually possible in the design of these multiple implant flaps to spare the papillae of the adjacent teeth. One of the main goals of utilizing an apically positioned flap is to preserve, or increase, the amount of keratinized tissue buccal to the fixture(s). The more the crestal incision is positioned towards the palatal/lingual the more keratinized tissue is moved apically and buccally to the implant(s). In the mandible we are usually more limited in moving our incision towards the lingual, since the amount of keratinization of the edentulous areas is reduced and there is no real advantage in completely depriving the lingual side of gingiva to slide it buccally. In the maxilla we find a greater source of keratinized tissue in the palatal vault. When the crestal incision is then pushed more towards the palatal

side, more bone may be left exposed in this area; techniques have been described by Tinti & Parma-Benfenati (2002) and by Nemcovsky et al. (1999) to obtain tissue from the remaining palatal mucosa to cover the osseous exposure.

In this regard the author of this chapter often finds that the thickness of the palate is enough to start splitting the flap at the cresto-palatal incision level, leaving a protective periosteal layer bound to the bone palatal to the implants (Figs. 16.58–16.60).

When the crestal incision falls within the confines of the implant head(s), the remaining portion of the platform is exposed by a semilunar incision (Fig. 16.61).

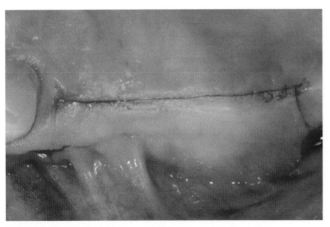

Figure 16.58 A crestopalatal incision is placed to uncover three maxillary implants.

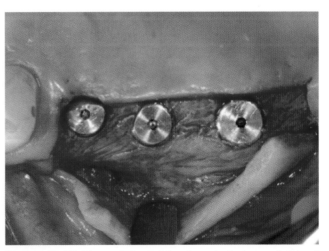

Figure 16.59 The splitting of the flap starts immediately at the level of the crestopalatal incision, leaving the inter-implant periosteum in place. A slight semilunar incision is done to expose the mesial implant further.

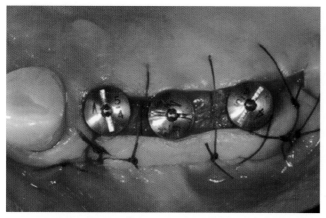

Figure 16.60 The flap is apically positioned with periosteal single interrupted sutures. A crossed-sling suture is used to obtain a tighter adaptation of the keratinized tissue buccally to the distal implant. A standard 4.1-mm diameter temporary healing abutment is placed on the distal fixture that has a 5-mm diameter according to the platform-switching concept.

It is advisable in designing the cresto-palatal split thickness flap to overextend it in the mesio-distal direction (Fig. 16.60). The wider transverse diameter of the buccal convexity of the maxillary alveolar process, compared to the smaller transverse diameter of the palatal concavity of the alveolar process, tends to increase the mesio-distal width of the vestibular recipient bed onto which the palatal mucosa is apically and buccally moved. Not taking this into consideration could result in a coronal pedicle narrower than its recipient bed, and thus not properly covering the mesio-distal extension of the implant(s). This problem becomes even more significant if we keep the two vertical releasing incisions divergent towards the vestibule rather than parallel to each other.

Once the healing abutments have been seated and checked for proper positioning on the implant platforms, suturing begins. The stabilization of the flap in its new apical and buccal position

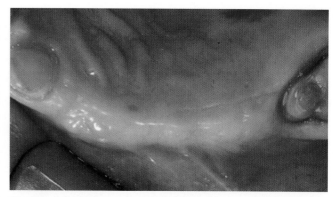

Figure 16.62 Pre-operative view of an area where four implants were previously placed.

is greatly enhanced by the presence of the buccal periosteal layer, onto which the sutures are anchored. Usually single interrupted sutures or external vertical or horizontal mattress are utilized to close up the wound. When a single flap is reflected (e.g., a single buccal flap) a mixed suture technique that combines either a single interrupted suture or an external vertical mattress on the flap side and an internal horizontal mattress on the opposite side can be used to help keep the designed flap more apical and adherent to the osseous crest (Figs. 16.56 & 16.61B).

This approach can be further modified using the palatal mucosa as a source of little pedicles that are interproximally rotated, in a similar fashion to that originally described by Pallacci & Ericsson (2001). This usually speeds up the healing of the interproximal areas, which can then be molded by the anatomical emergence profiles of the abutment/crown complexes (Figs. 16.62–16.66).

Sometimes, in the posterior maxilla in conjunction with the apically repositioned flap, the thickness of the residual tissue palatal to the implants needs further thinning. This is accomplished in a fashion similar to what we do during periodontal pocket elimination surgery, with the goal of reducing the final palatal peri-implant probing depth (Fig. 16.67).

Figure 16.61 (A) Pre-operative view of the area where three implants were previously placed. (B) Implants were uncovered via an apically positioned buccal flap and palatal semilunar incisions. View of the sutured buccal flap. (C) Healing of the tissue. Note the good quality and quantity of the peri-implant mucosa. (D) Occlusal view of the definitive screw-retained implant-supported restoration.

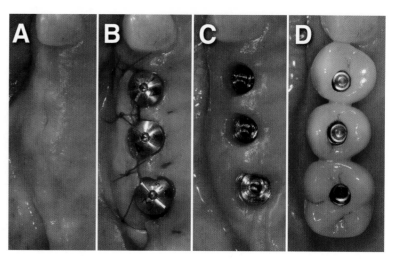

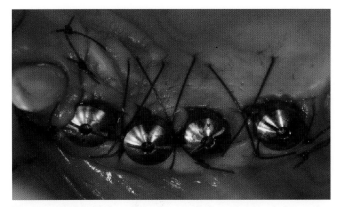

Figure 16.63 Little triangular pedicles obtained from the mucosa palatal to the three last distal implants are interproximally rotated and stabilized in position by crossed horizontal external mattress sutures.

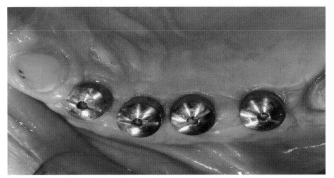

Figure 16.64 Postoperative healing of the area 4 weeks after the uncovering. There is good maturation of the inter-implant tissues.

BUCCALLY POSITIONED ENVELOPE FLAP

This approach, designed by Smukler et al. (2003a,b), represents in its simplicity of execution a brilliant attempt to surgically idealize the peri-implant soft tissue profiles (Figs. 16.68–16.70).

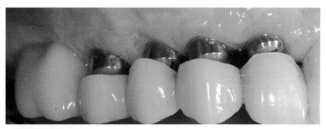

Figure 16.65 Buccal view of postoperative healing of the area 4 weeks after the uncovering. There is good maturation of the interproximal areas and an adequate scalloped soft tissue profile. The provisional restoration was modified to make room for the temporary healing abutments.

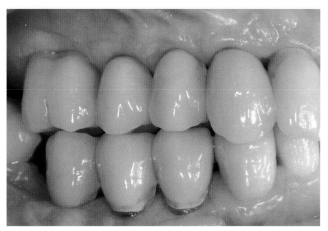

Figure 16.66 Final implant-supported restoration in place. Note the harmonious soft tissue profiles.

It is usually indicated for single implants in the esthetic zone, although it can be utilized for multiple implants. A blade no. 15C is used to draw a straight incision from the palatal line angle of the mesial dental element to the palatal line angle of the distal one. A full-thickness envelope flap is raised towards the buccal after intrasulcular incisions are placed on each adjacent tooth.

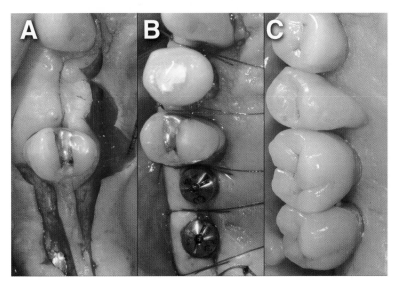

Figure 16.67 (A) View of the incision of the area where three implants were previously placed; the first in position of the first bicuspid and the remaining two distal to the natural second bicuspid. The palatal flap is shortened and thinned to reduce final peri-implant probing depths and to eradicate a periodontal pocket palatal to the natural tooth (B) External vertical mattress sutures are used to position the incised tissue at the osseous crest. A screw-retained temporary crown was placed on the mesial implant while healing abutments were used for the distal ones. (C) Healing of the tissues. Note the good quality and quantity of the peri-implant mucosa.

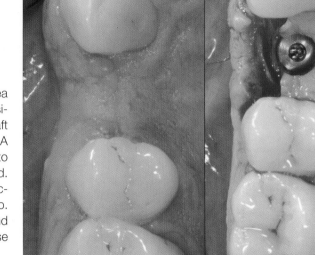

Figure 16.68 (A) Pre-operative view of the area to be uncovered. Together with a buccally positioned envelope flap, a connective tissue graft is planned to plump up the buccal ridge. (B) A straight incision is designed from the canine to the premolar. No vertical incisions are placed. A full thickness flap is reflected and a connective tissue graft is slid under the buccal flap. Note the palatal donor area already sutured and the semilunar incision performed to fully expose the implant platform.

No vertical releasing incisions should be utilized. The buccal portion of the cover screw is now visible and a semilunar palatal incision is placed to fully expose the implant platform and allow for proper seating of the healing abutment or, even better, of the provisional restoration when available.

The flap is held standing in its buccal position by the healing abutment or provisional crown. Two horizontal internal mattress sutures are placed at the base of each papilla to stabilize the flap and avoid compression on the papillary areas. With a fresh blade no. 15C the buccal gingival scallop is then designed, making sure the proposed buccal gingival margin is drawn at a more coronal level than the ones on the adjacent teeth. This is done to produce an excess of buccal tissue, which can be fine-tuned by the anatomically designed temporary restoration, knowing that a certain degree of apical recession is normally expected (Grunder 2000).

A two-stage surgical approach similar to the one described earlier has been proposed by Tinti & Benfenati (2002) to obtain papillae between multiple implants in the esthetic zone.

In order for these techniques to be successfully performed it is important to pre-operatively evaluate the amount of buccal keratinized tissue that is available. If the area presents with a lack of buccal gingival tissue there is a risk of further reducing this amount. Under this circumstance either a different approach (e.g., apically positioned flap) should be selected or the

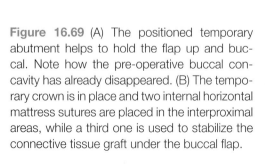
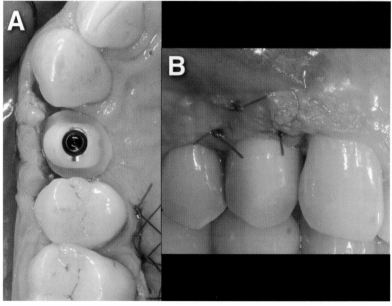

Figure 16.69 (A) The positioned temporary abutment helps to hold the flap up and buccal. Note how the pre-operative buccal concavity has already disappeared. (B) The temporary crown is in place and two internal horizontal mattress sutures are placed in the interproximal areas, while a third one is used to stabilize the connective tissue graft under the buccal flap.

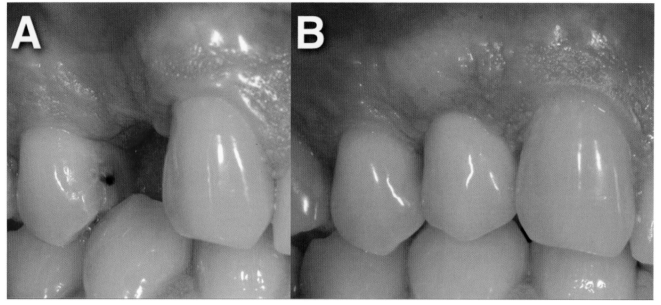

Figure 16.70 (A) Pre-operative view of the edentulous area. Note the good amount of keratinized mucosa but also the marked buccal concavity present after the loss of the natural dental element. (B) After surgical uncovering of the implant the ideal quality and quantity of tissue are present.

keratinized tissue (e.g., free gingival graft) should be augmented before proceeding with the buccally positioned envelope flap.

BUCCALLY POSITIONED SCALLOPED FLAP FOR MULTIPLE IMPLANTS

This surgical approach has been designed to uncover multiple implants when there is an esthetic expectation that needs to be fulfilled. The second-stage surgery under these circumstances must be preceded by osseous reconstructive maneuvers (with or without concomitant soft tissue grafting) that idealize the tridimensional volume of the area either before or at the time of implant placement. Often, as a consequence of the previous regenerative procedures, the shape of the edentulous area is ideal but there may be alterations in the normal position of the mucogingival junction that result in a more coronal position.

At the second surgical stage the profile at the top of the ridge should be flat, drawing a straight line from the distal papilla of the mesial dental element to the mesial papilla of the distal tooth; if this is the case the soft tissue at the top of the ridge will become the peak of the interimplant papilla, thus recreating an harmonious anatomy.

The key step in flap design is therefore not to incise at the summit of the ridge, thus preserving the future interimplant papillary height. The second important concept, to be followed while incising the area, is related to the determination of the mucogingival junction that becomes the apical boundary of the band of

keratinized mucosa within which the scalpel designs the flap. To properly draw the incision it is important to move between the top of the ridge and the mucogingival line without impinging on them and while attempting to include at least 2 mm of keratinized mucosa in the flap.

The incision is of partial thickness and properly scalloped to obtain better flap adaptation around the implant collar and permit a better closure of the interimplant areas.

When available, the use of a provisional prosthesis to anticipate the desired final mucosal margin can guide the surgeon in correct flap festooning, always keeping in mind the two untouchable coronal and apical limits within which the incision must be placed (Figs. 16.71–16.73).

CONNECTIVE TISSUE GRAFT

A subepithelial connective tissue graft (Langer & Calagna 1980) can be used during stage one surgery to build up the ridge volume in a bucco-lingual and/or an apico-coronal direction. At uncovering, the placement of the healing screw or the temporary crown precludes the use of a connective tissue graft to plump up the area coronally. During second-stage surgery it is possible to utilize such a graft to augment the bucco-lingual volume of the ridge, creating the illusion of a root prominence, increasing the gingival thickness, and generally improving the final esthetic result (Figs. 16.74–16.78). For certain edentulous spaces, where major contour deficiencies are present, soft tissue grafting can be repeated several times (stage one, stage

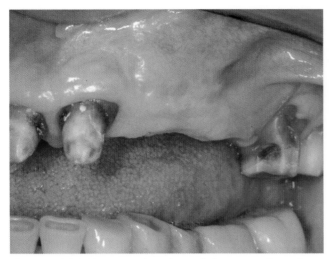

Figure 16.71 Pre-operative view of the area where three implants were already placed in the canine and two bicuspids positions. The missing lateral was planned to be cantilevered off the canine. A guided bone regeneration was also performed at the time of implant placement, creating an almost ideal flat ridge profile.

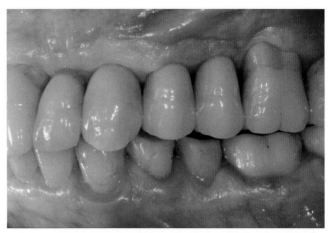

Figure 16.73 Final implant-supported prosthesis is in place. Note the good quantity and quality of the peri-implant mucosa surrounding the canine and the bicuspids.

two, and also between the two stages) to achieve the desired result. Multiple grafts can be obtained within the same surgical procedure by several donor sites and strategically positioned where most needed.

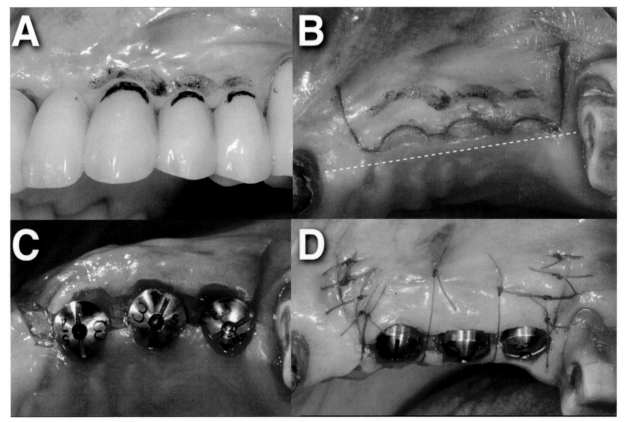

Figure 16.72 (A) The provisional prosthesis is repositioned into place and the use of a surgical marker highlights the ideal desired final position of the gingival margin. (B) The marked line can not be incised where it is due to its proximity to the muco-gingival junction, and it is copied in its design by the actual incision line, which is shifted about 2 mm more coronally without reaching the summit of the ridge (hyphenated line). (C) View of the scalloped partial thickness buccal flap and the palatal semilunar incisions. Healing abutments are in place. (D) Sutures are in place. Note the good amount of keratinized mucosa sutured buccal to the healing abutments and how the inter-implant mucosa has not been incised during the procedure.

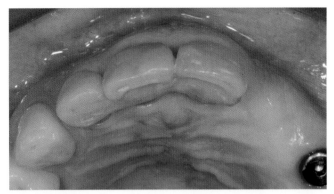

Figure 16.74 A single implant was previously added to those already present to replace the missing left maxillary canine. The plan in the area was to position an implant bridge with the missing lateral cantilevered off the canine. Note at the time of uncovering the flat buccal soft tissue profile in the missing canine area and the slightly concave tissue profile in the lateral incisor location.

The recipient site is prepared in a similar fashion to what is required for traditional periodontal root coverage procedures. It is always preferable to design the incision by splitting the periostium in order to maintain the osseous periosteal coverage as an additional source of nourishment for the subepithelial connective tissue graft. However, when grafting the area during implant placement (stage one) it is accepted to place the graft between the osseous surface, denuded by a full thickness flap, and the flap itself.

During uncovering procedures a no. 15C blade is used to draw a straight, or slightly scalloped, crestal incision that continues in the interproximal and buccal sulcus of each adjacent tooth. A partial-thickness buccal flap is obtained by severing the periostium well beyond the muco-gingival line, paying attention

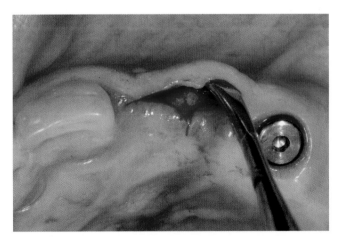

Figure 16.75 A partial thickness "envelope" flap is designed where the volumetric increase of the soft tissue is desired. Note the small periosteal elevator lifting the scalloped buccal flap.

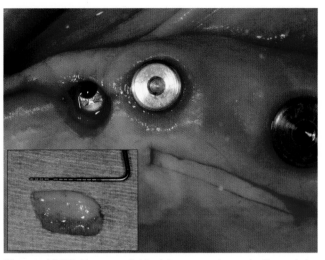

Figure 16.76 Two parallel incisions are drawn in the palate: the coronal one at a 90° angle to the underlying osseous plane and the apical one (usually the bleeding one) almost parallel to the bone plane. Note the procured connective tissue graft in the lower left corner box.

not to perforate the vestibular tissue. Vertical releasing incisions are not needed. A semilunar incision is designed to uncover the palatal portion of the cover screw from the remaining covering tissue, to allow the seating of the prosthetic components. The palatal mucosa surrounding the implant platform is usually not reflected unless its thickness exceeds 4 mm. When this is the case, reflecting the palatal tissue allows it to be thinned, while simultaneously collecting the connective tissue graft from the inner portion of the palatal flap. The graft is sutured buccally to the periostium using single interrupted resorbable 5-0 gut or 6-0 Vycril sutures. The collected connective tissue can also be stabilized by suturing it to the inner aspect of the vestibular flap with an internal horizontal mattress suture, always keeping the knot on the outer buccal surface of the flap.

When the thinning of the mucosa immediately palatal to the implant is not needed, the donor site is prepared as originally described by Bruno (1994). Always in the palate, 2–3 mm below the gingival margin of the adjacent posterior teeth, a first straight incision is placed at 90° to the teeth and down to the bone.

A second, more apical incision, parallel to the first one, is then drawn, this time keeping the blade parallel to the long axis of the teeth (Fig. 16.76). The distance between the two incision lines determines the thickness of the graft; the closer the space between the parallel lines the thinner the graft and vice versa. Once the palatal incisions are placed a periosteal elevator is introduced to the most coronal incision to dissect a full thickness wedge of connective tissue. To fully detach the graft two additional lateral incisions are placed, entering with a no. 15C blade between the two parallel lines, first mesial and then

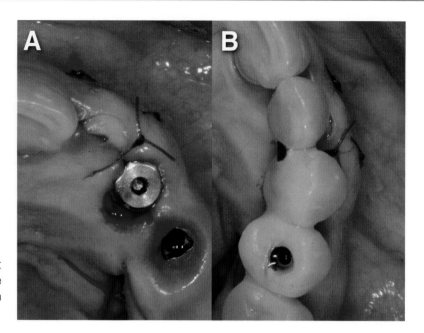

Figure 16.77 (A) The connective tissue graft is in place and suturing is completed. (B) The screw-retained temporary bridge is seated in position.

distal to the wedge of tissue. In order to facilitate the execution of these two lateral incisions it is useful to slightly overextend the two initial parallel incision lines to obtain more space to enter and maneuver the blade.

After removal of the soft tissue from the donor site, the remaining epithelial layer is dissected from the graft, while the palatal wound is closed using either a suspended horizontal crossed suture or a crossed horizontal external mattress suture.

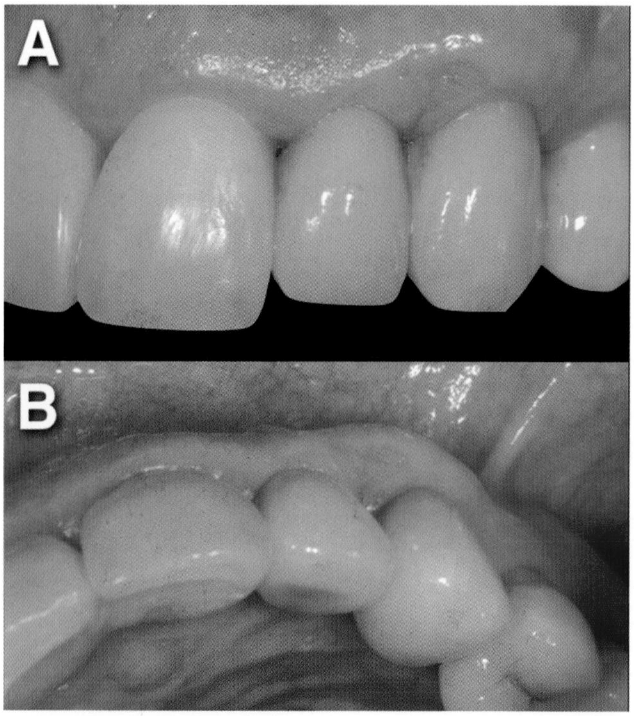

The connective tissue graft may also be obtained in the retro-molar tuberosity area in a fashion similar to the procedure used when designing a distal wedge during periodontal surgery.

Once the graft has been sutured into place, the previously raised buccal envelope flap is closed on top of it by horizontal or vertical internal mattress suturing.

The connective tissue graft approach is an extremely versatile procedure. It is often executed in association with an apically positioned flap or a buccally positioned envelope flap.

MODIFIED ROLL TECHNIQUE

This relatively easy procedure is used in the maxilla to obtain a localized increase in the soft tissue volume buccal to the implant (Abrams 1980; Scharf & Tarnow 1992; Israelson & Plemons 1993; Barone et al. 1999) (Figs. 16.79–16.84). The first straight crestal incision is kept palatal to the head of the implant, orienting the scalpel, to obtain a long external bevel that extends down to the bone. Two vertical releasing incisions are drawn starting from the palatine bevel, sparing the interproximal papillae, and extending passed the muco-gingival line. A small periosteal elevator, which enters from the vertical releasing incisions, is then used to carefully reflect buccally a full-thickness flap together with its palatine "tail". This usually requires some delicacy in order to avoid tearing and damaging the palatine tail connected to the buccal flap. The epithelial layer of the flap, palatal to the head of the fixture, is then sliced off with a sharp no. 15C blade. The palatal portion of the long-tailed flap is then rolled and tucked under the buccal flap.

Figure 16.78 (A) Frontal view of the definitive restoration. (B) Occlusal view of the definitive restoration. Note the good quality and quantity of the peri-implant mucosa.

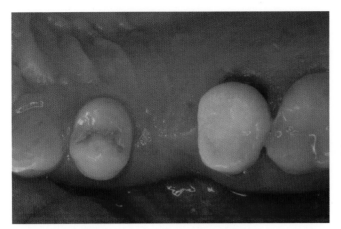

Figure 16.79 Pre-operative view of the area. The mesiobuccal root of the first maxillary molar, now wearing a provisional crown, was previously resected for periodontal reasons. An implant was placed in the edentulous space of the missing second premolar. Note the buccal concavity.

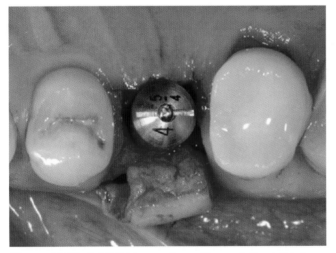

Figure 16.80 A full-thickness flap with a palatine tail is buccally reflected.

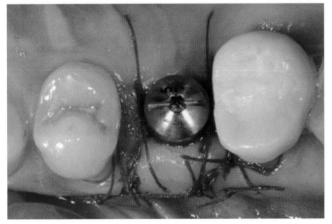

Figure 16.81 Suturing is completed. There is an increase in the buccal volume of tissue (compare with Fig. 16.79).

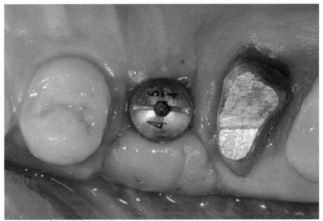

Figure 16.82 Early healing in the area.

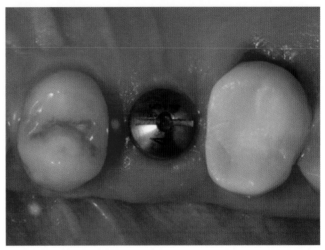

Figure 16.83 Mature healing in the area. A soft tissue convexity visible buccal to the implant simulates a root prominence.

Sometimes the thickness of the flap is such that it becomes difficult to tuck the most palatal portion of it under the buccal flap. To make this easier the tissue can be slightly thined (decreasing the amount of volumetric increase that will be eventually obtained in the area) or a horizontal partial-thickness releasing incision can be positioned, right where the tissue should bend under the vestibular flap.

A horizontal internal mattress suture is used to keep the rolled tissue in position. After seating of the healing abutment additional single interrupted sutures are used to close the verticals, and external vertical mattress sutures can be placed to properly adapt the rolled flap to the osseous ridge (Figs. 16.85–16.89).

FREE GINGIVAL GRAFT

This approach still represents the gold standard in augmenting the quantity of keratinized tissue surrounding a fixture (Alpert

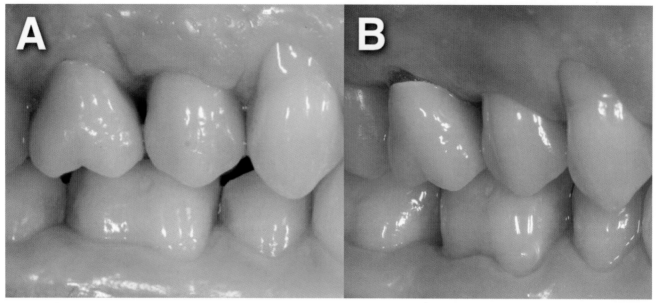

Figure 16.84 (A) Completed case with final restorations on the root resected maxillary molar and on the premolar implant. (B) After 8 years the gingival tissue has slightly receded on the crowned molar and on the first premolar while stable mucosal tissue is noticeable buccal to the implant. Note how the previously visible scar distal to the implant has faded away with time.

1994) (Figs. 16.90–16.93). The surgical technique does not substantially differentiate from what happens around natural teeth (Sullivan & Atkins 1968).

With a no. 15C blade a recipient periosteal bed is designed buccal to the implant, which has been previously exposed with a punch-blade approach. In preparing the recipient bed it is important to completely dissect all the elastic and muscular fibers. Failure to do this will result in an island of still movable albeit keratinized tissue. To increase the firmness of the adherence of the free gingival graft to the underlying recipient bed the periostium is additionally scored down to the bone with a scalpel to expose little strips of osseous tissue in the recipient area (Dordick et al. 1976).

Once the recipient area has been prepared the donor site is chosen. Potential donor zones are the palatal mucosa between the first molar and the first premolar, other edentulous ridges, the tuberosity area, and sometimes the posterior maxillary buccal ridge, provided there is enough keratinized tissue. The latter area is the one that usually offers the tissue that blends best, allowing for a good esthetic result.

When grafting around an implant it is advisable to surgically collect a slightly thicker layer of epithelialized connective tissue as compared to grafting around a natural tooth. It has been hypothesized that with an increased thickness of the connective tissue portion of the graft its capillary system is better preserved (Holbrook & Ochsenbein 1983; Miller 1987). A faster

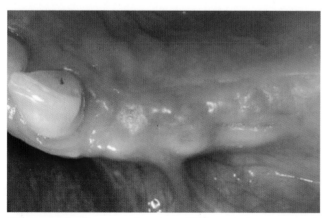

Figure 16.85 Pre-operative view of the area to be uncovered. Three implants are buried under the tissue. The thickness of the edentulous ridge is reduced.

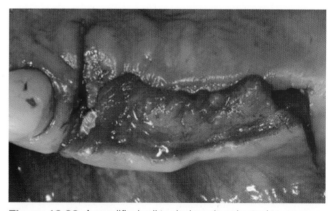

Figure 16.86 A modified roll technique is selected to uncover the three implants. To simplify the procedure, a vertical palatal release is placed, and the flap with its palatine connective tissue tail is buccally reflected.

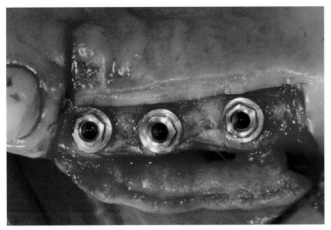

Figure 16.87 The tail is tucked under the buccal flap to increase the buccal thickness of tissue while simultaneously reducing the thickness of the palatal tissue. With this technique, the volume of tissue is increased where it is most needed for aesthetics, and the peri-implant palatal probings are reduced.

activation of this more intact vascular network, in a thicker graft, may compensate for a reduction in the plasmic circulation originating from the peri-implant recipient bed (Sullivan & Atkins 1968; Miller 1987).

The absence of the periodontal ligament, the presence of a more cortical quality to the bone, and the reduced presence of vessels in the peri-implant soft tissues all combine to reduce nourishment to the graft, which may necrotize and eventually slough off.

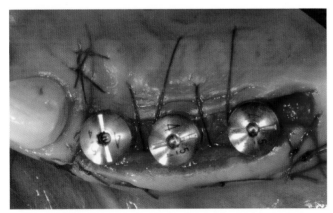

Figure 16.88 While single interrupted sutures close the vertical-releasing incisions, combined internal (buccally) and external (palatally) mattress sutures close the interimplant areas. As a result, the buccal flap is held up against the healing abutments while compressing the connective tissue tail, and the thinned palatal flap is compressed down against the palatal bone. This kind of suturing will produce a ramp in the soft tissue from the buccal side toward the palate.

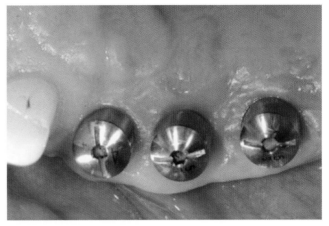

Figure 16.89 Final healing of the area. Note the increase in the volume of soft tissue buccal to the implants and the thin tissue palatal to the fixtures (compare with Fig. 16.85).

To further increase the chances of graft survival additional factors must be considered: the concordance between the dimension of the recipient site and the graft itself, an adequate hemostasis between the graft and its periosteal bed, and a tight adaptation between the graft and the underlying periostium. The proper adaptation of the free gingival graft to the recipient area is provided and maintained by the suturing technique, which should ensure a light compression of the surgical area while stabilizing the graft in place (Holbrook & Ochsenbein 1983).

XENOGRAFTS TO IMPROVE PERI-IMPLANT KERATINIZATION

In spite of the great efficacy of free gingival grafting a considerable site morbidity in the donor area has been reported (Griffin et al. 2006).

The need for a second surgical area from which to harvest the epithelialized connective tissue graft increases the length of the procedure, exposes the patient to a mild hemorrhagic risk due to the proximity of the palatal artery, and increases postoperative discomfort.

To overcome these issues the potential use of xenografts as a substitute to palatal grafts to augment the amount of keratinized tissue around implants and teeth has been investigated in a randomized prospective clinical trial (Sanz et al. 2009) (Figs. 16.94–16.97).

Twenty patients were investigated over 6 months, comparing connective tissue grafting to the use of a porcine collagen matrix, and it was concluded that the tridimensional matrix was not statistically different from the autologous tissue (Sanz et al. 2009). The increase in keratinization produced by both techniques at 6 months amounted to around 2.5 mm, with a

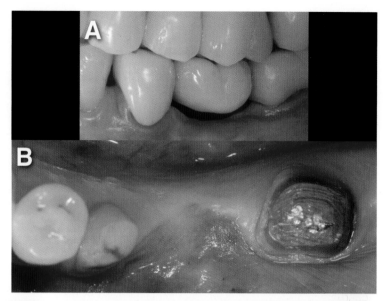

Figure 16.90 (A) Preoperative buccal view, at the time of second stage surgery, of an implant previously placed to replace the first mandibular molar. (B) The occlusal view of the area after removal of the provisional restoration shows a lack of keratinized mucosa buccal to the implant.

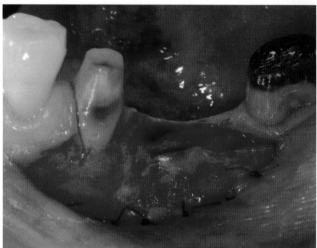

Figure 16.91 In preparation for a free gingival graft a periosteal bed is prepared buccal to the implant and the natural bicuspid.

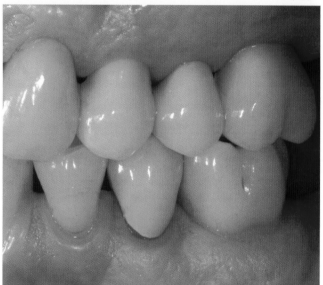

Figure 16.93 Final restorations after 5 years. Note the ideal quality and quantity of keratinized tissue present.

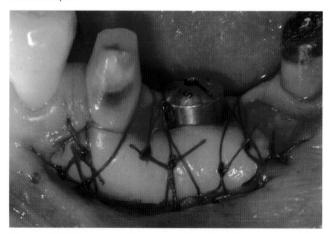

Figure 16.92 A palatally procured epithelial and connective tissue graft is sutured in position with single and suspended 5-0 Vicryl sutures.

graft contraction of 60% for the connective tissue and 67% for the collagen matrix at 1 month. In terms of tissue recession the behavior was similar and so was the tissue blending. The porcine matrix statistically reduced patient discomfort and total surgery time when compared to autologous grafting.

Similar conclusions were reported in a subsequent study on the same porcine collagenous matrix preformed around the teeth of five patients treated in a split-mouth design (Nevins et al. 2011). In this pilot case series study plaque and gingival indices were evaluated together with probing pocket depth, gingival recession and the amount of attached gingiva at both baseline and 12-month follow-up. Each patient was treated with the collagenous matrix on one side of the mouth while an autologous graft was placed on the other side. In addition to the

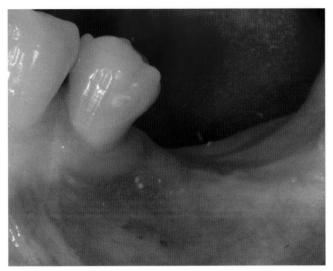

Figure 16.94 Pre-operative buccal view at the time of second-stage surgery to uncover two implants distal to the first mandibular premolar. Note the lack of keratinized mucosa in the edentulous area.

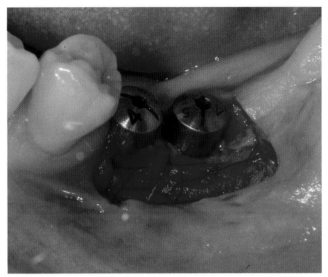

Figure 16.96 The porcine collagenous matrix has been sutured with 6-0 Vicryl on a periosteal bed in a similar fashion of a free gingival graft.

clinical evaluation, biopsies were procured from both surgical sites at about 13 weeks healing time. A clinically significant increase in the amount of attached gingiva was measured in both cases (2.3 ± 1.1 mm for the xenograft vs 3.1 ± 0.6 mm for the autograft) with no statistically significant differences for any of the evaluated clinical parameters when comparing autologous grafting to the xenograft. The treated patients favored the use of the collagen matrix to avoid a second surgical site and the evaluated blending of the graft was superior for the matrix. The collected histology did not show any difference between the two grafts. No signs of inflammatory reactions were ever

reported and a mature connective tissue covered by ortho-keratinized epithelium characterized the biopsy sections.

The same group of authors carried out a randomized controlled split-mouth study on six patients to investigate the efficacy of another extracellular matrix membrane of xenogeneic origin for gingival augumentation (Nevins et al. 2010b) (Figs. 16.98–16.101).

This study, similar to the previous one, evaluated the xenograft both clinically and histologically in comparison to an autograft used as a control within the same patient. The clinical data (plaque index, gingival index, probing depth, recession, and amount of keratinized gingiva) were collected at baseline and

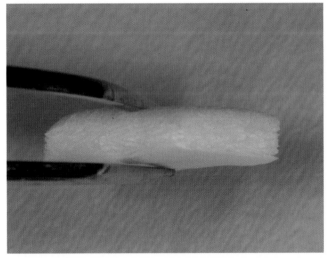

Figure 16.95 A xenogeneic bio-absorbable collagen matrix (Mucograft®, Geistlich Pharma AG) is chosen for the uncovering procedure.

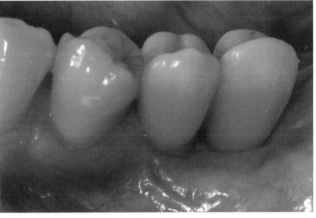

Figure 16.97 Definitive implant-supported crowns are in place and a sufficient amount of immobile keratinized mucosa is now present buccal to the implants.

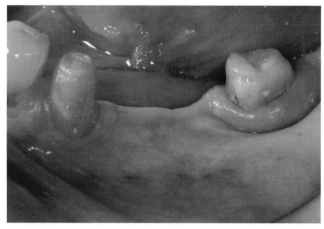

Figure 16.98 Pre-operative buccal view at the time of second-stage surgery to uncover two implants previously placed in the edentulous area. Note the lack of keratinized mucosa in the edentulous area.

after 13 weeks of healing when a soft tissue biopsy was also obtained.

No statistically significant difference was reported for any of the clinical measures, except for the amount of keratinized gingiva, where the mean change postoperatively was 5.3 ± 1.3 mm for the autograft vs 2.6 ± 1.1 mm for the xenograft ($P = 0.002$). In spite of this difference it must be highlighted how this other porcine matrix was also effective in increasing the amount of keratinization with an average value (around 2.5 mm) that is in line with what was reported in the previously quoted studies. Once again the blending of the collagenous matrix membrane was better than for the autologous tissue, with a concomitant reduction in patient discomfort since they did not have to undergo the palatal harvest.

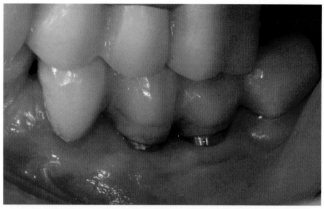

Figure 16.100 Healing of the area. Provisional restoration is still in place. Note the augmented quantity of keratinized tissue buccal to the natural premolar and to the two implants.

The histologic evaluation conducted revealed mature connective tissue covered by orthokeratinized epithelium without differences between test and controls. No inflammatory reaction was visible in any of the tested samples and at 13 weeks no remnants of the collagenous matrix could be seen.

The first clinical study performed specifically on implants to test the behavior of a xenogeneic bio-absorbable collagen matrix was published in 2012 (Lorenzo et al. 2012). This parallel, randomized clinical trial evaluated 6-month results, in terms of keratinized mucosal augmentation, when utilizing the matrix in comparison to the free connective tissue autograft. A total of 24 patients with at least one implant serving as an abutment of implant-supported restorations and with minimal or no keratinized mucosa (≤1 mm) were investigated. During surgery, following preparation of the recipient vascular bed, a free connective tissue graft was allocated in the control group while a

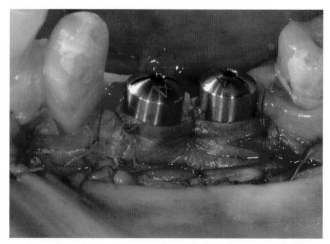

Figure 16.99 A xenogeneic bio-absorbable porcine collagen matrix (Dynamatrix®, Keystone Dental) is sutured in the recipient periosteal bed, buccal to the second premolar and to the two dental implants.

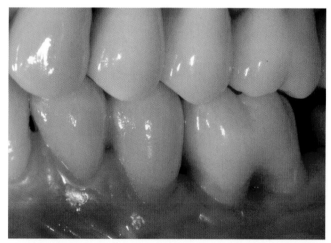

Figure 16.101 After 3 years the final restorations are in position. The two implants support the first mandibular molar. Note the stable sufficient amount of keratinized mucosa buccal to the implants and the increased quantity of keratinized tissue on the second premolar (compare with Fig. 16.98).

Mucograft® collagenous matrix was used for the test group. At the 6-month evaluation the autologous graft produced a mean width of keratinized tissue of 2.75 mm (SD 1.5 mm) while the xenograft produced 2.8 mm (SD 0.4 mm) of mucosal keratinization. The difference is not statistically significant. The aesthetic performance, in terms of color and tissue blending, between tests and controls was indistinguishable by blinded evaluators. Although not statistically significant, the patients treated with the collagen matrix reported less pain. The measured surgical time was significantly lower for the matrix than for the autologous graft.

The results of the investigations confirmed the data previously published by Sanz et al. (2009) using the same biomaterial. In this specific study the xenograft behaved similarly to the autograft, with values similar to what was previously reported of 2.5–3 mm of keratinization measured postoperatively. It should be noted that the collagenous matrix employed in this research produced results, in terms of keratinization, that were more consistent than for the autologous graft, as exemplified by the reduced standard deviation value (0.4 mm vs 1.5 mm).

The really intriguing question when evaluating the clinical behavior of these matrices, which are capable of increasing the amount of keratinized mucosa, relates to the biological mechanism underlying this phenomenon. Current knowledge postulates that only gingival connective tissue, or connective tissue from the periodontium, has the capacity to induce keratinized epithelium (Karring et al. 1975) and therefore it appears logical to assume that the xenogeneic matrices probably function according to different biological pathways.

According to the hypothesis (Nevins et al. 2010b), while the blood vessels and the fibroblast invade the matrix, which acts as a permeable scaffold, the epithelial layer that overlies the xenograft originates from the surrounding epithelium. If that is so, it could be beneficial to have these collagenous scaffolds surrounded by as much keratinized tissue as possible. The surgical approach that will be described is based on this assumption.

The recipient site is prepared as previously reported in the section on free gingival graft, with the only significant difference being that a minimal band of keratinized mucosa (1 mm at least) is dissected through a split-thickness flap from the top of the ridge to be sutured at the apical base of the periosteal bed. The lingual side of the implant is usually uncovered with a semilunar incision. Once isolated, the periosteal recipient site bordered mostly by keratinized tissue, a properly pre-shaped piece of collagen of xenogeneic origin is sutured in place in a similar manner to what was described for autologous tissue.

In cases where there is a complete lack of keratinized mucosa at the time of implant uncovering the preference of this author is still to choose an autologous graft that can be substituted by a xenograft when there is a minimal amount (usually around 1 mm) of keratinization present in the area.

PAPILLA REGENERATION TECHNIQUES

As already discussed at the beginning of this chapter, there seem to be limitations to what it is possible to achieve in terms of re-creation of the lost papillary tissue (Tarnow et al. 2003). This is especially true for multiple implant rehabilitations. Several techniques have been designed in an attempt to surgically idealize the shape of the lost papilla (Salama et al. 1995; Adriaenssens et al. 1999; Palacci & Ericsson 2001; Tinti & Benfenati 2002; Smukler et al. 2003a & b). The reader is referred to these references for descriptions of the different surgical procedures.

CONCLUSION

It is important to keep in mind that, aside from the selected surgical approach for the uncovering, the final presence of good papillae and gingival scallop surrounding the implant is dependent on several other factors. Between these factors the author would like to close this chapter by emphasizing the importance of a properly designed prosthetic restoration (Smukler et al. 2003a & b).

The carefully customized anatomical shape of the temporary prosthesis should start molding the surrounding peri-implant soft tissues as soon as possible. It is important to evaluate the degree of maturation of the soft tissue when exerting strategically located pressure to idealize the peri-implant gingival profiles. A mature thick tissue can withstand higher degrees of pressures compared to a still healing thin tissue, which could react to the push with a sudden undesirable recession.

Once it is believed that the proper prosthetic sculpting of the gingiva has been achieved the final restoration can be positioned. It is the responsibility of the surgeon to provide the prosthodontist with the right quality and quantity of both hard and soft tissues to start the prosthetic molding process. In achieving the final desired result continuous and harmonious interaction between several caregivers (surgeon, prosthodontist, dental technician, hygienist) and the patient is of utmost importance.

At the conclusion of active treatment a carefully designed individual maintenance program will ensure the long-term success of this team achievement.

REFERENCES

Abrahamsson, I., Berglundh, T., & Lindhe, J. (1997) The mucosal barrier following abutment dis/reconnection. An experimental study in dogs. *Journal of Clinical Periodontology* 24(8), 568–572.

Abrahamsson, I., Zitzmann, N.U., Berglundh, T., Linder, E., Wennerberg, A., & Lindhe, J. (2002) The mucosal attachment to titanium implants with different surface characteristics: an experimental study in dogs. *Journal of Clinical Periodontology* 29(5), 448–455.

Abrams, L. (1980) Augmentation of the deformed residual edentulous ridge for fixed prosthesis. *Compendium of Continuing Education in Dentistry* 1, 205–214.

Adell, R., Lekholm, U., Rockler, B., & Branemark, P.I. (1981) A 15-year study of osseointegrated implants in the treatment of the edentulous jaw. *International Journal of Oral Surgery* 10(6), 387–416.

Adibrad, M., Shahabuei, M., & Sahabi, M. (2009) Significance of the width of keratinized mucosa on the health status of the supporting tissue around implants supporting overdentures. *Journal of Oral Implantology* 35(5), 232–237.

Adriaenssens, P., Hermans, M., Ingber, A., Prestipino, V., Daelemans, P., & Malevez, C. (1999) Palatal sliding strip flap: soft tissue management to restore maxillary anterior esthetics at stage 2 surgery: a clinical report. *International Journal of Oral Maxillofacial Implants* 14(1), 30–36.

Albrektsson, T., & Zarb, G.A. (1993) current interpretations of the osseointegrated response: Clinical significance. *International Journal of Prosthodontics* 6, 95–105.

Alpert, A. (1994) A rationale for attached gingiva at the soft-tissue/implant interface: esthetic and functional dictates. *Compendium of Continuing Education in Dentistry* 15, 356–366.

Apse, P., Zarb, G.A., Schmitt, A., & Lewis, D.W. (1991) The longitudinal effectiveness of osseointegrated dental implants. The Toronto Study: peri-implant mucosal response. *The International Journal of Periodontics and Restorative Dentistry* 11(2), 94–111.

Astrand, P., Engquist, B., Dahlgren, S., Grondahl, K., Engquist, E., & Feldmann, H. (2004) Astra Tech and Branemark system implants: a 5-year prospective study of marginal bone reactions. *Clinical Oral Implants Research* 15(4), 413–420.

Atieh M.A., Ibrahim, H.M., & Atieh, A.H. (2010) Platform switching for marginal bone preservation around dental implants: a systematic review and meta-analysis. *Journal of Periodontology* 81(10), 1350–1366.

Bakaeen, L., Quinlan, P., Schoolfield, J., Lang, N.P., & Cochran, D.L. (2009) The biologic width around titanium implants: histometric analysis of the implantogingival junction around immediately and early loaded implants. *The International Journal of Periodontics and Restorative Dentistry* 29(3), 297–305.

Barone, R., Clauser, C., & Prato, G.P. (1999) Localized soft tissue ridge augmentation at phase 2 implant surgery: a case report. *The International Journal of Periodontics and Restorative Dentistry* 19(2), 141–145.

Barros, R.R., Novaes Jr A.B., Muglia, V.A., Iezzi, G., & Piattelli, A. (2010) Influence of interimplant distances and placement depth on peri-implant bone remodeling of adjacent and immediately loaded Morse cone connection implants: a histomorphometric study in dogs. *Clinical Oral Implants Research* 21(4), 371–378.

Bashutski, J.D., & Wang, H.L. (2007) Common implant esthetic complications. *Implant Dentistry* 16, 340–348.

Becker, W., Ochsenbein, C., Tibbetts, L., & Becker, B.E. (1997) Alveolar bone anatomic profiles as measured from dry skulls. Clinical ramifications. *Journal of Clinical Periodontology* 24(10), 727–731.

Bengazi, F., Wennström, J.L., & Lekholm, U. (1996) Recession of the soft tissue margin at oral implants. A 2-year longitudinal prospective study. *Clinical Oral Implants Research* 7(4), 303–310.

Benic, G.I., Mokti, M., Chen, C.J., Weber, H.P., Hammerle, C.H.F., & Gallucci, G.O. (2012) Dimensions of buccal bone and mucosa at immediately placed implants after 7 years: a clinical and cone beam computed tomography study. *Clinical Oral Implants Research* 23, 560–566.

Berglundh, T., & Lindhe, J. (1996) Dimension of the periimplant mucosa. Biological width revisited. *Journal of Clinical Periodontology* 23(10), 971–973.

Berglundh, T., Lindhe, J., Ericsson, I., Marinello, C.P., Liljenberg, B., & Thomsen, P. (1991) The soft tissue barrier at implants and teeth. *Clinical Oral Implants Research* 2(2), 81–90.

Berglundh, T., Lindhe, J., Jonsson, K., & Ericsson, I. (1994) The topography of the vascular systems in the periodontal and peri-implant tissues in the dog. *Journal of Clinical Periodontology* 21(3), 189–193.

Block, M.S., & Kent, J.N. (1990) Factors associated with soft and hard tissue compromise of endosseous implants. *Journal of Oral Maxillofacial Surgery* 48, 1153–1160.

Bouri, A. Jr, Bissada, N., Al-Zahrani, M.S., Faddoul, F., & Nouneh, I. (2008) Width of keratinized gingiva and the health status of the supporting tissue around dental implants. *International Journal of Oral Maxillofacial Implants* 23, 323–326.

Boynuegry, D., Nemli, S.K., & Kasko, Y.A. (2013) Significance of keratinized mucosa around dental implants: a prospective comparative study. *Clinical Oral Implants Research* 24, 928–933.

Bruno, J.F. (1994) Connective tissue graft technique assuring wide root coverage. *The International Journal of Periodontics and Restorative Dentistry* 14(2), 126–137.

Burkhardt, R., Joss, A., & Lang, N.P. (2008) Soft tissue dehiscence coverage around endosseous implants: a prospective cohort study. *Clinical Oral Implants Research* 19(5), 451–457.

Buser, D., Martin, W., & Belser, U.C. (2004) Optimizing esthetics for implant restorations in the anterior maxilla: Anatomic and surgical considerations. *International Journal of Oral Maxillofacial Implants* 19(Suppl), 43–61.

Buser, D., Halbritter, S., Hart, C., Bornstein, M.M., Grutter, L., Chappuis, V., & Belser, U.C. (2009) Early implant placement with simultaneous guided bone regeneration following single tooth extraction in the esthetic zone: 12-month results of a prospective study with 20 consecutive patients. *Journal of Periodontology* 80, 152–162.

Buser, D., Wittneben, J., Bornstein, M.M., Grutter, L., Chappuis, V., & Belser, U.C. (2011) Stability of contour augmentation and esthetic outcomes of implant supported single crowns in the esthetic zone: 3-year results of a prospective study with early implant placement postextraction. *Journal of Periodontology* 82, 342–349.

Cairo, F., Pagliaro, U., & Nieri, M. (2008) Soft tissue management at implant sites. *Journal of Clinical Periodontology* 35(Suppl 8), 163–167.

Canullo, L., Bignozzi, I., Cochetto, R., Cristalli, M.P., & Ianello, G. (2010a) Immediate positioning of a definitive abutment versus repeated abutment replacements in post-extractive implants: 3-year follow up of a randomised multicentre clinical trial. *European Journal of Oral Implantology* 3(4), 285–296.

Canullo, L., Fedele, G.R., Iannello, G., & Jepsen, S. (2010b) Platform switching and marginal bone-level alterations: the results of a randomized-controlled trial. *Clinical Oral Implants Research* 21(1), 115–121.

Cardaropoli, G., Lekholm, U., & Wennström, J.L. (2006) Tissue alterations at implant-supported single-tooth replacements: a 1-year prospective clinical study. *Clinical Oral Implants Research* 17(2), 165–171.

Chang, M., Wennström, J.L., Odman, P., & Andersson, B. (1999) Implant supported single-tooth replacements compared to contralateral natural teeth. Crown and soft tissue dimensions. *Clinical Oral Implants Research* 10(3), 185–194.

Choquet, V., Hermans, M., Adriaenssens, P., Daelemans, P., Tarnow, D.P., & Malevez, C. (2001) Clinical and radiographic evaluation of the papilla level adjacent to single-tooth dental implants. A retrospective study in the maxillary anterior region. *Journal of Periodontology* 72(10), 1364–1371.

Chow, Y.C., & Wang, H.L. (2010) Factors and techniques influencing peri-implant papillae. *Implant Dentistry* 19(3), 208–219.

Chung, D.M., Oh, T.J., Shotwell, J.L., Misch, C.E., & Wang, H.L. (2006) Significance of keratinized mucosa in maintenance of dental implants with different surfaces. *Journal of Periodontology* 77, 1410–1420.

Costa, F.O., Takenaka-Martinez, S., Cota, L.O., Ferreira, S.D., Silva, G.L., & Costa, J.E. (2012) Peri-implant disease in subjects with and without preventive maintenance: a 5-year follow-up. *Journal of Clinical Periodontology* 39(2), 173–181.

Cosyn, J., & De Rouck, T. (2009) Aesthetic outcome of single-tooth implant restorations following early implant placement and guided bone regeneration: crown and soft tissue dimension compared with controlateral teeth. *Clinical Oral Implants Research* 20, 1063–1069.

Degidi, M., Novaes, A.B. Jr, Nardi, D., & Piattelli, A. (2008) Outcome analysis of immediately placed, immediately restored implants in the esthetic area: the clinical relevance of different interimplant distances. *Journal of Periodontology* 79(6), 1056–1061.

Degidi, M., Perrotti, V., Shibli, J.A., Novaes, A.B., Piattelli, A., & Iezzi, G. (2011a) Equicrestal and subcrestal dental implants: a histologic and histomorphometric evaluation of nine retrieved human implants. *Journal of Periodontology* 82(5), 708–715.

Degidi, M., Nardi, D., & Piattelli, A. (2011b) One abutment at one time: Non removal of an immediate abutment and its effect on bone healing around subcrestal tapered implants. *Clinical Oral Implants Research* 22, 1303–1307.

Degidi, M., Piattelli, A., Scarano, A., Shibli, J.A., & Iezzi, G. (2012) Peri-implant collagen fibers around human cone Morse connection implants under polarized light: a report of three cases. *The International Journal of Periodontics and Restorative Dentistry* 32(3), 323–328.

De Sanctis, M., Vignoletti, F., Discepoli, N., Muñoz, F., & Sanz, M. (2010) Immediate implants at fresh extraction sockets: an experimental study in the beagle dog comparing four different implant systems. Soft tissue findings. *Journal of Clinical Periodontology* 37(8), 769–776.

Dharmar, S., Yoshida, K., Adachi, Y., Kishi, M., Okuda, K., & Sekine, H. (1994) Subgingival microbial flora associated with brånemark implants. *International Journal of Oral Maxillofacial Implants* 9(3), 314–318.

Dordick, B., Coslet, J.G., & Seibert, J.S. (1976) Clinical evaluation of free autogenous gingival grafts placed on alveolar bone. Part II. Coverage of nonpathologic dehiscences and fenestrations. *Journal of Periodontology* 47(10), 568–573.

Ericsson, I., Nilner, K., Klinge, B., & Glantz, P.O. (1996) Radiographical and histological characteristics of submerged and nonsubmerged titanium implants. An experimental study in the Labrador dog. *Clinical Oral Implants Research* 7(1), 20–26.

Esposito, M., Grousovin, M.G., Maghaireh, H., Coulthard, P., & Worthington, H.V. (2007) Interventions for replacing missing teeth: management of soft tissue for dental implants. *Cochrane Database Systematic Review* 18(3), CD006697.

Esposito, M., Maghaireh, H., Grusovin, M.G., Ziounas, I., & Worthington, H.V. (2012) Soft tissue management for dental implants: What are the most effective techniques? *A Cochrane Systematic Review. European Journal of Oral Implantology* 5(3), 221–238.

Ferreira, S.D., Silva, G.L., Cortelli, J.R., Costa, J.E., & Costa, F.O. (2006) Prevalence and risk variables for peri-implant disease in Brazilian subjects. *Journal of Clinical Periodontology* 33(12), 929–935.

Friedmann, A., Strietzel, F.P., Maretzki, B., Pitaru, S., & Bernimoulin, J.P. (2002) Histological assessment of augmented jaw bone utilizing a new collagen barrier membrane compared to a standard barrier membrane to protect a granular bone substitute material. *Clinical Oral Implants Research* 13(6), 587–594.

Gallucci, G.O., Grutter, L., Chuang, S.K., & Belser, U.C. (2011) Dimensional changes of periimplant soft tissue over 2 years with single-implant crowns in the anterior maxilla. *Journal of Clinical Periodontology* 38, 293–299.

Garber, D.A., & Belser, U.C. (1995) Restoration-driven implant placement with restoration-generated site development. *Compendium of Continuing Education in Dentistry* 16(8), 796, 798–802, 804.

Garber, D.A., Salama, M.A., & Salama, H. (2001) Immediate total tooth replacement. *Compendium of Continuing Education in Dentistry* 22(3), 210–216, 218.

Gargiulo, A.W., Wentz, F.M., & Orban, B. (1961) Dimensions and relations of the dento-gingival junction in humans. *Journal of Periodontology* 32, 261–267.

Gastaldo, J.F., Cury, P.R., & Sendyk, W.R. (2004) Effect of the vertical and horizontal distances between adjacent implants and between a tooth and an implant on the incidence of interproximal papilla. *Journal of Periodontology* 75(9), 1242–1246.

Glauser, R., Schupbach, P., Gottlow, J., & Hammerle, C.H.F. (2005) Peri-implant soft tissue barrier at experimental one piece mini implants with different surface topography in humans: A light microscopic overview and histometric analysis. *Clinical Implant Dentistry-Related Research* 7(Suppl 1), s44–s51.

Goldman, H.M., & Cohen, D.W. (1980) *Periodontal Therapy*, 6th edn. C.V. Mosby, St Louis, pp. 670–677.

Grandi, T., Guazzi, P., Samarani, R., & Garuti, G. (2012) Immediate positioning of definitive abutments versus repeated abutment replacements in immediately loaded implants: effects on bone healing at the 1-year follow up of a multicenter randomised controlled trial. *European Journal of Oral Implantology* 5(1), 9–16.

Griffin, T.J., Cheung, W.S., Zavras, A.I., & Damoulis, P.D. (2006) Postoperative complications following gingival augmentation procedures. *Journal of Periodontology* 77, 2070–2090.

Grunder, U. (2000) Stability of the mucosal topography around single-tooth implants and adjacent teeth: 1-year results. *The

International Journal of Periodontics and Restorative Dentistry 20(1), 11–17.

Grunder, U., Gracis, S., & Capelli, M. (2005) Influence of the 3-D bone-to-implant relationship on esthetics. *The International Journal of Periodontics and Restorative Dentistry* 25(2), 113–119.

Harris, R.J. (1994) The connective tissue with partial thickness double pedicle graft: the results of 100 consecutively-treated defects. *Journal of Periodontology* 65(5), 448–461.

Hermann, J.S., Cochran, D.L., Nummikoski, P.V., & Buser, D. (1997) Crestal bone changes around titanium implants. A radiographic evaluation of unloaded nonsubmerged and submerged implants in the canine mandible. *Journal of Periodontology* 68(11), 1117–1130.

Hermann, J.S., Buser, D., Schenk, R.K., & Cochran, D.L. (2000) Crestal bone changes around titanium implants. A histometric evaluation of unloaded non-submerged and submerged implants in the canine mandible. *Journal of Periodontology* 71(9), 1412–1424.

Hermann, J.S., Buser, D., Schenk, R.K., Schoolfield, J.D., & Cochran, D.L. (2001) Biologic width around one- and two-piece titanium implants. *Clinical Oral Implants Research* 12(6), 559–571.

Hertel, R.C., Blijdorp, P.A., Kalk, W., & Baker, D.L. (1994) Stage II surgical techniques in endosseous implantation. *International Journal of Oral Maxillofacial Implants* 9, 273–278.

Holbrook, T., & Ochsenbein, C. (1983) Complete coverage of the denuded root surface with a one-stage gingival graft. *The International Journal of Periodontics and Restorative Dentistry* 3(3), 8–27.

Holt, R.L., Rosenberg, M.M., Zinser, P.J., & Ganeles, J. (2002) A concept for a biologically derived, parabolic implant design. *The International Journal of Periodontics and Restorative Dentistry* 22(5), 473–481.

Hurzeler, M.B., & Weng, D. (1996) Periimplant tissue management: optimal timing for an aesthetic result. *Practical Periodontics Aesthetics Dentistry* 8(9), 857–869; quiz 869.

Iglhaut, G., Becker, K., Golubovic, V., Schliephake, H., & Mihatovic, I. (2013) The impact of dis/reconnection of laser microgrooved and machined implant abutments on soft and hard tissue healing. *Clinical Oral Implants Research* 24, 391–397.

Israelson, H., & Plemons, J.M. (1993) Dental implants, regenerative techniques, and periodontal plastic surgery to restore maxillary anterior esthetics. *International Journal of Oral Maxillofacial Implants* 8(5), 555–561.

Jemt, T., Ahlberg, G., Henriksson, K., & Bondevik, O. (2006) Changes of anterior clinical crown height in patients provided with single-implant restorations after more than 15 years of follow-up. *International Journal of Prosthodontics* 19(5), 455–461.

Jovanovic, S.A., & Nevins, M. (1995) Bone formation utilizing titanium-reinforced barrier membranes. *The International Journal of Periodontics and Restorative Dentistry* 15(1), 56–69.

Kan, J.Y., Rungcharassaeng, K., Umezu, K., & Kois, J.C. (2003) Dimensions of peri-implant mucosa: an evaluation of maxillary anterior single implants in humans. *Journal of Periodontology* 74(4), 557–562.

Karring, T., Lang, N.P., & Löe, H. (1975) The role of gingival connective tissue in determining epithelial differentiation. *Journal of Periodontal Research* 10(1), 1–11.

Kazor, C.E., Al-Shammari, K., Sarment, D.P., Misch, C.E., & Wang, H.L. (2004) Implant plastic surgery: a review and rationale. *Journal of Oral Implantology* 30(4), 240–254.

Kim, B.S., Kim, Y.K., Yun, P.Y., Yi, Y.J., Lee, H.J., Kim, S.G., & Son, J.S. (2009) Evaluation of peri-implant tissue response according to the presence of keratinized mucosa. *Oral Surg Oral Med Oral Pathol Oral Radiol Endod.* 107, e24–e28.

Kois, J.C. (1996) The restorative-periodontal interface: biological parameters. *Periodontology 2000* 11, 29–38.

Koldsland, O.C., Scheie, A.A., & Aass, A.M. (2010) Prevalence of peri-implantitis related to severity of the disease with different degrees of bone loss. *Journal of Periodontology* 81(2), 231–238.

Kon, S., Caffesse, R.G., Castelli, W.A., & Nasjleti, C.E. (1984) Vertical releasing incisions for flap design: clinical and histological study in monkeys. *The International Journal of Periodontics and Restorative Dentistry* 4(1), 48–57.

Koutouzis, T., Koutouzis, G., Gadalla, H., & Neiva, R. (2013) The effect of healing abutment reconnection and disconnection on soft and hard peri-implant tissue: A short-term randomized controlled clinical trial. *International Journal of Oral Maxillofacial Implants* 28, 807–814.

Landi, L., & Sabatucci, D. (2001) Plastic surgery at the time of membrane removal around mandibular endosseous implants: a modified technique for implant uncovering. *The International Journal of Periodontics and Restorative Dentistry* 21(3), 280–287.

Lang, N.P., Wilson, T.G., & Corbet, E.F. (2000) Biological complications with dental implants: their prevention, diagnosis and treatment. *Clinical Oral Implants Research* 11(Suppl 1), 146–155.

Langer, B., & Calagna, L. (1980) The subepithelial connective tissue graft. *Journal of Prosthetic Dentistry* 44(4), 363–367.

Langer, B., & Langer, L. (1985) Subepithelial connective tissue graft technique for root coverage. *Journal of Periodontology* 56(12), 715–720.

Lekholm, U., Sennerby, L., Roos, J., & Becker, W. (1996) Soft tissue and marginal bone conditions at osseointegrated implants that have exposed threads: A 5-year retrospective study. *International Journal of Oral Maxillofacial Implants* 11, 599–604.

Linkevicius, T., & Apse, P. (2008) Biologic width around implants. An evidence-based review. *Stomatologija, Baltic Dental and Maxillofacial Journal* 10, 27–35.

Listgarten, M.A., Lang, N.P., Schroeder, H.E., & Schroeder, A. (1991) Periodontal tissues and their counterparts around endosseous implants. *Clinical Oral Implants Research* 2(3), 1–19.

Lorenzo, R., García, V., Orsini, M., Martin, C., & Sanz, M. (2012) Clinical efficacy of a xenogeneic collagen matrix in augmenting keratinized mucosa around implants: a randomized controlled prospective clinical trial. *Clinical Oral Implants Research* 23(3), 316–324.

Maynard, J.G. Jr, & Wilson, R.D. (1979) Physiologic dimensions of the periodontium significant to the restorative dentist. *Journal of Periodontology* 50(4), 170–174.

Miller, P.D. Jr. (1987) Root coverage with the free gingival graft. Factors associated with incomplete coverage. *Journal of Periodontology* 58(10), 674–681.

Moon, I.S., Berglundh, T., Abrahamsson, I., Linder, E., & Lindhe, J. (1999) The barrier between the keratinized mucosa and the dental implant. An experimental study in the dog. *Journal of Clinical Periodontology* 26(10), 658–663.

Mormann, W., & Ciancio, S.G. (1977) Blood supply of human gingiva following periodontal surgery. A fluorescein angiographic study. *Journal of Periodontology* 48(11), 681–692.

Moy, P.K., Weinlaender, M., & Kenney, E.B. (1989) Soft-tissue modifications of surgical techniques for placement and uncovering of osseointegrated implants. *Dent Clin North Am*. 33(4), 665–681.

Muller, H.P., & Eger, T. (2002) Masticatory mucosa and periodontal phenotype: a review. *The International Journal of Periodontics and Restorative Dentistry* 22(2), 172–183.

Nelson, S.W. (1987) The subpedicle connective tissue graft. A bilaminar reconstructive procedure for the coverage of denuded root surfaces. *Journal of Periodontology* 58(2), 95–102.

Nemcovsky, C.E., Artzi, Z., & Moses, O. (1999) Rotated split palatal flap for soft tissue primary coverage over extraction sites with immediate implant placement. Description of the surgical procedure and clinical results. *Journal of Periodontology* 70(8), 926–934.

Nemcovsky, C.E., Moses, O., Artzi, Z., & Gelernter, I. (2000) Clinical coverage of dehiscence defects in immediate implant procedures: three surgical modalities to achieve primary soft tissue closure. *International Journal of Oral Maxillofacial Implants* 15(6), 843–852.

Nevins, M., & Mellonig, J.T. (1998) *Implant therapy. Clinical approaches and evidence of success*. Quintessence Publishing Co. Inc., p. 227.

Nevins, M., Nevins, M.L., Camelo, M., Boyesen, J.L., & Kim, D.M. (2008) Human histologic evidence of a connective tissue attachment to a dental implant. *The International Journal of Periodontics and Restorative Dentistry* 28(2), 111–121.

Nevins, M., Kim, D.M., Jun, S.H., Guze, K., Schupbach, P., & Nevins, M.L. (2010a) Histologic evidence of a connective tissue attachment to laser microgrooved abutments: a canine study. *The International Journal of Periodontics and Restorative Dentistry* 30(3), 245–255.

Nevins, M., Nevins, M.L., Camelo, M., Camelo, J.M., Schupbach, P., & Kim, D.M. (2010b) The clinical efficacy of DynaMatrix extracellular membrane in augmenting keratinized tissue. *The International Journal of Periodontics and Restorative Dentistry* 30(2), 151–161.

Nevins, M., Nevins, M.L., Kim, S.W., Schupbach, P., & Kim, D.M. (2011) The use of mucograft collagen matrix to augment the zone of keratinized tissue around teeth: a pilot study. *The International Journal of Periodontics and Restorative Dentistry* 31(4), 367–373.

Nevins, M., Camelo, M., Nevins, M.L., Schupbach, P., & Kim, D.M. (2012) Connective tissue attachment to laser-microgrooved abutments: a human histologic case report. *The International Journal of Periodontics and Restorative Dentistry* 32(4), 385–392.

Nisapakultorn, K., Suphanantachat, S., Silkosessak, O., & Rattanamongkolgul, S. (2010) Factors affecting soft tissue level around anterior maxillary single-tooth implants. *Clinical Oral Implants Research* 21, 662–670.

Novaes, A.B. Jr,, De Oliveira, R.R., Muglia, V.A., Papalexiou, V., & Taba, M. Jr (2006) The effects of interimplant distances on papilla formation and crestal resorption in implants with a morse cone connection and a platform switch: a histomorphometric study in dogs. *Journal of Periodontology* 77, 1839–1849.

Novaes, A.B. Jr, Barros, R.R., Muglia, V.A., & Borges, G.J. (2009) Influence of interimplant distance and placement depth on papilla formation and crestal resorption: a clinical and radiographic study in dogs. *Journal of Oral Implantology* 35(1), 18–27.

Olsson, M., Lindhe, J., & Marinello, C.P. (1993) On the relationship between crown form and clinical features of the gingiva in adolescents. *Journal of Clinical Periodontology* 20(8), 570–577.

Palacci, P., & Ericsson, I. (2001) *Esthetic Implant Dentistry: Soft & Hard Tissue*. Quintessence Publishing Co. Inc.

Piattelli, A., Scarano, A., Piattelli, M., Bertolai, R., & Panzoni, E. (1997) Histologic aspects of the bone and soft tissues surrounding three titanium non-submerged plasma-sprayed implants retrieved at autopsy: a case report. *Journal of Periodontology* 68(7), 694–700.

Pjetursson, B.E., Tan, K., Lang, N.P., Bragger, U., Egger, M., & Zwahlen, M. (2004) A systematic review of the survival and complication rates of fixed partial dentures (FPDs) after an observation period of at least 5 years. *Clinical Oral Implants Research* 15(6), 625–642.

Puchades-Roman, L., Palmer, R.M., Palmer, P.J., Howe, L.C., Ide, M., & Wilson, R.F. (2000) A clinical, radiographic, and microbiologic comparison of Astra Tech and Branemark single tooth implants. *Clinical Implant Dentistry-Related Research* 2(2), 78–84.

Rodriguez, X., Vela, X., Mendez, V., Segalà, M., Calvo-Guirado, J., & Tarnow, D.P. (2013) The effect of abutment dis/reconnections on peri-implant bone resorption: A radiologic study of platform-switched and non-platform-switched implants placed in animals. *Clinical Oral Implants Research* 24, 305–311.

Rompen, E. (2012) The impact of the type and configuration of abutments and their (repeated) removal on the attachment level and marginal bone. *European Journal of Oral Implantology* 5(Suppl), S83–S90.

Rompen, E., Touati, B., & Van Dooren, E. (2003) Factors influencing marginal tissue remodeling around implants. *Practical Procedings in Aesthetic Dentistry* 15(10), 754–757, 759, 761.

Rompen, E., Domken, O., Degidi, M., Pontes, A.E., & Piattelli, A. (2006) The effect of material characteristics, of surface topography and of implant components and connections on soft tissue integration: a literature review. *Clinical Oral Implants Research* 17(Suppl2), 55–67.

Roos-Jansaker, A.M., Renvert, H., Lindahl, C., & Renvert, S. (2006) Nine to fourteen-year follow-up of implant treatment. Part III: factors associated with periimplant lesions. *Journal of Clinical Periodontology* 33(4), 296–301.

Rosenquist, B. (1997) A comparison of various methods of soft tissue management following the immediate placement of implants into extraction sockets. *International Journal of Oral Maxillofacial Implants* 12(1), 43–51.

Saadoun, A.P. (1997) The key to peri-implant esthetics: hard- and soft-tissue management. *Dental Implantology Update* 8(6), 41–46.

Saadoun, A.P., & LeGall, M. (1992) Implant positioning for periodontal, functional, and aesthetic results. *Practical Periodontics in Aesthetic Dentistry* 4(7), 43–54.

Salama, H., Salama, M., Garber, D., & Adar, P. (1995) Developing optimal peri-implant papillae within the esthetic zone: guided soft tissue augmentation. *Journal of Esthetic Dentistry* 7(3), 125–129.

Salama, H., Salama, M.A., Garber, D., & Adar, P. (1998) The interproximal height of bone: a guidepost to predictable aesthetic strategies and soft tissue contours in anterior tooth replacement. *Pract Periodontics Aesthet Dent* 10(9), 1131–1141.

Sanz, M., Lorenzo, R., Aranda, J.J., Martin, C., & Orsini, M. (2009) Clinical evaluation of a new collagen matrix (Mucograft prototype) to enhance the width of keratinized tissue in patients with fixed prosthetic restorations: a randomized prospective clinical trial *Journal of Clinical Periodontology* 36(10), 868–876.

Scarano, A., Assenza, B., Piattelli, M., Thams, U., San Roman, F., Favero, G.A., & Piattelli, A. (2004) Interimplant distance and crestal bone resorption: a histologic study in the canine mandible. *Clin Implant Dent Relat Res* 6(3), 150–156.

Scharf, D.R., & Tarnow, D.P. (1992) Modified roll technique for localized alveolar ridge augmentation. *The International Journal of Periodontics and Restorative Dentistry* 12(5), 415–425.

Schierano, G., Ramieri, G., Cortese, M., Aimetti, M., & Preti, G. (2004) Organization of the connective tissue barrier around long-term loaded implant abutments in man. *Clinical Oral Implants Research* 15(1), 66–72.

Schmidlin, K., Schnell, N., Steiner, S., Salvi, G.E., Pjetursson, B., Matuliene, G., Zwahlen, M., Bragger, U., & Lang, N.P. (2010) Complication and failure rates in patients treated for chronic periodontitis and restored with single crowns on teeth and/or implants. *Clinical Oral Implants Research* 21(5), 550–557.

Schneider, D., Grunder, U., Ender, A., Hammerle, C.H.F., & Jung, R.E. (2011) Volume gain and stability of periimplant soft tissue following bone and soft tissue augmentation: 1-year results from a prospective cohort study. *Clinical Oral Implants Research* 22, 28–37.

Schroeder, A., Van der Zypen, E., Stich, H., & Sutter, F. (1981) The reactions of bone, connective tissue, and epithelium to endosteal implants with titanium-sprayed surfaces. *Journal of Maxillofacial Surgery* 9(1), 15–25.

Schrott, R.A., Jimenez, M., Hwang, J.W., Fiorellini, J., & Weber, H.P. (2009) Five year evaluation of the influence of keratinized mucosa on periimplant soft tissue health and stability around implants supporting full arch mandibular fixed prosthesis. *Clinical Oral Implants Research* 20, 1170–1177.

Schupbach, P., & Glauser, R. (2007) The defense architecture of the human periimplant mucosa: a histological study. *Journal of Prosthetic Dentistry* 97(6 Suppl), S15–S25.

Sclar, A.J. (2003) *Soft tissue and esthetic considerations in implant therapy*. Quintessence Publishing Co., Inc., pp. 142–143.

Silverstein, L.H., Kurtzman, D., Garnick, J.J., Trager, P.S., & Waters, P.K. (1994) Connective tissue grafting for improved implant esthetics: clinical technique. *Implant Dent* 3(4), 231–234.

Simion, M., Trisi, P., & Piattelli, A. (1994) Vertical ridge augmentation using a membrane technique associated with osseointegrated implants. *The International Journal of Periodontics and Restorative Dentistry* 14(6), 496–511.

Siqueira, S. Jr, Pimentel, S.P., Alves, R.V., Sendyk, W., & Cury, P.R. (2013) Evaluation of the effects of buccal-palatal bone width on the incidence and height of the interproximal papilla between adjacent implants in esthetic areas. *Journal of Periodontology* 84(2), 170–175.

Small, P.N., & Tarnow, D.P. (2000) Gingival recession around implants: a 1-year longitudinal prospective study. *International Journal of Oral Maxillofacial Implants* 15(4), 527–532.

Smukler, H., & Chaibi, M. (1997) Periodontal and dental considerations in clinical crown extension: a rational basis for treatment. *The International Journal of Periodontics and Restorative Dentistry* 17(5), 464–477.

Smukler, H., & Dreyer, C.J. (1969) Principal fibres of the periodontium. *Journal of Periodontal Research* 4(1), 19–25.

Smukler, H., Castellucci, F., & Capri, D. (2003a) The role of the implant housing in obtaining aesthetics: generation of peri-implant gingivae and papillae-Part 1. *Pract Proceed Aesthet Dent* 15(2), 141–149.

Smukler, H., Castellucci, F., & Capri, D. (2003b) The role of the implant housing in obtaining aesthetics: Part 2. Customizing the peri-implant soft tissue. *Pract Proceed Aesthet Dent* 15(6), 487–490.

Soadoun, A.P., & Touati, B. (2007) Soft tissue recession around implants: Is it still unavoidable? Part II. *Pract Proceed Aesthet Dent* 19(2), 81–87.

Spray, J.R., Black, C.G., Morris, H.F., & Ochi, S. (2000) The influence of bone thickness on facial marginal bone response: Stage I placement through stage 3 uncovering. *Ann Periodontol* 5, 119–128.

Staffileno, H., Levy, S., & Gargiulo, A. (1966) Histologic study of cellular mobilization and repair following a periosteal retention operation via split thickness mucogingival flap surgery. *Journal of Periodontology* 37(2), 117–131.

Sullivan, H.C., & Atkins, J.H. (1968) Free autogenous gingival grafts. 1. Principles of successful grafting. *Periodontics* 6(1), 5–13.

Tarnow, D.P., Magner, A.W., & Fletcher, P. (1992) The effect of the distance from the contact point to the crest of bone on the presence or absence of the interproximal dental papilla. *Journal of Periodontology* 63(12), 995–996.

Tarnow, D.P., Cho, S.C., & Wallace, S.S. (2000) The effect of inter-implant distance on the height of inter-implant bone crest. *Journal of Periodontology* 71(4), 546–549.

Tarnow, D., Elian, N., Fletcher, P., Froum, S., Magner, A., Cho, S.C., Salama, M., Salama, H., & Garber, D.A. (2003) Vertical distance from the crest of bone to the height of the interproximal papilla between adjacent implants. *Journal of Periodontology* 74(12), 1785–1788.

ten Bruggenkate, C.M., Krekeler, G., Van der Kwast, W.A.M., & Oosterbeek, H.S. (1991) Palatal mucosal grafts for oral implant devices. *Oral Surg Oral Med Oral Pathol* 72, 154–158.

Teughels, W., Merheb, J., & Quirynen, M. (2009) Critical horizontal dimensions of interproximal and buccal bone around implants for optimal aesthetic outcomes: a systematic review. *Clinical Oral Implants Research* 20(Suppl 4), 134–145.

Tinti, C., & Benfenati, S.P. (2002) The ramp mattress suture: a new suturing technique combined with a surgical procedure to obtain papillae between implants in the buccal area. *The International Journal of Periodontics and Restorative Dentistry* 22(1), 63–69.

Tinti, C., & Parma-Benfenati, S. (1995) Coronally positioned palatal sliding flap. *The International Journal of Periodontics and Restorative Dentistry* 15(3), 298–310.

Todescan, F.F., Pustiglioni, F.E., Imbronito, A.V., Albrektsson, T., & Gioso, M. (2002) Influence of the microgap in the peri-implant hard and soft tissues: a histomorphometric study in dogs. *International Journal of Oral Maxillofacial Implants* 17(4), 467–472.

Triaca, A., Minoretti, R., Merli, M., & Merz, B. (2001) Periosteoplasty for soft tissue closure and augmentation in preprosthetic surgery: a surgical report. *International Journal of Oral Maxillofacial Implants* 16(6), 851–856.

Tymstra, N., Raghoebar, G.M., Vissink, A., Den Hartog, L., Stellingsma, K., & Meijer, H.J. (2011) Treatment outcome of two adjacent implant crowns with different implant platform designs in the aesthetic zone: a 1-year randomized clinical trial. *Journal of Clinical Periodontology* 38(1), 74–85.

Vacek, J.S., Gher, M.E., Assad, D.A., Richardson, A.C., & Giambarresi, L.I. (1994) The dimensions of the human dentogingival junction. *The*

International Journal of Periodontics and Restorative Dentistry 14(2), 154–165.

Vignoletti, F., De Sanctis, M., Berglundh, T., Abrahamsson, I., & Sanz, M. (2009) Early healing of implants placed into fresh extraction sockets: an experimental study in the beagle dog. III: Soft tissue findings. *Journal of Clinical Periodontology* 36(12), 1059–1066.

Warrer, K., Buser, D., Lang, N.P., & Karring, T. (1995) Plaque-induced peri-implantitis in the presence or absence of keratinized mucosa. An experimental study in monkeys. *Clinical Oral Implants Research* 6(3), 131–138.

Weisgold, A.S., Arnoux, J.P., & Lu, J. (1997) Single-tooth anterior implant: a world of caution. Part I. *Journal of Esthetic Dentistry* 9(5), 225–233.

Weng, D., Nagata, M.J., Bell, M., Bosco, A.F., De Melo, L.G., & Richter, E.J. (2008) Influence of microgap location and configuration on the periimplant bone morphology in submerged implants. An experimental study in dogs. *Clinical Oral Implants Research* 19(11), 1141–1147.

Wennström, J., & Derks, J. (2012) Is there a need for keratinized mucosa around implants to maintain health and tissue stability? *Clinical Oral Implants Research* 23(Suppl 6), 136–146.

Wennstrom, J.L., Bengazi, F., & Lekholm, U. (1994) The influence of the masticatory mucosa on the peri-implant soft tissue condition. *Clinical Oral Implants Research* 5(1), 1–8.

Wöhrle, P.S. (2003) Nobel Perfect esthetic scalloped implant: rationale for a new design. *Clin Implant Dent Relat Res* 5(1), 64–73.

Zigdon, H., & Machtei, E.E. (2008) The dimensions of keratinized mucosa around implants affect clinical and immunological parameters. *Clinical Oral Implants Research* 19, 387–392.

Zitzmann, N.U., Naef, R., & Scharer, P. (1997) Resorbable versus non-resorbable membranes in combination with Bio-Oss for guided bone regeneration. *International Journal of Oral Maxillofacial Implants* 12(6), 844–852.

Zucchelli, G., Mele, M., Stefanini, M., Mazzotti, C., Marzadori, M., Montebugnoli, L., & De Sanctis, M. (2010) Patient morbidity and root coverage outcome after subepithelial connective tissue and de-epithelialized grafts: a comparative randomized-controlled clinical trial. *Journal of Clinical Periodontology* 37, 728–738.

Zucchelli, G., Mazzotti, C., Mounssif, I., Mele, M., Stefanini, M., & Montebugnoli, L. (2013) A novel surgical-prosthetic approach for soft tissue dehiscence coverage around single implant. *Clinical Oral Implants Research* 24, 957–962.

Chapter 17 Improving Patients' Smiles: Aesthetic Crown-Lengthening Procedure

Serge Dibart

HISTORY

There are two aspects to the crown-lengthening procedure: aesthetic and functional. In both cases the surgical procedure is aimed at reestablishing the biological width apically while exposing more tooth structure. The biological width is defined as the sum of the junctional epithelium and supracrestal connective tissue attachment (Cohen 1962).

Gargiulo et al. (1961), who measured the human dentogingival junction, found that the average space occupied by the sum of the junctional epithelium and the supracrestal connective tissue fibers is 2.04 mm. Violation of that space by restorations impinging on the biological width has been associated with gingival inflammation, discomfort, gingival recession, alveolar bone loss, pocket formation, and the like (Parma-Benfenati et al. 1985; Tarnow et al. 1986; Tal et al. 1989).

To have a harmonious and successful long-term restoration, Ingber et al. (1977) advocated 3 mm of sound supracrestal tooth structure between bone and prosthetic margins, which allows for the reformation of the biological width plus sulcus depth. This can be achieved surgically (crown lengthening) or orthodontically (forced eruption) or by a combination of both (Ingber 1976; Pontoriero et al. 1987; de Waal & Castellucci 1994).

INDICATIONS

- To improve the gummy smile of a patient with a high smile line

- To rehabilitate dentition that is compromised by the presence of extensive caries, short clinical crowns, traumatic injuries, or severe parafunctional habits

- To restore gingival health when the biological width has been violated by a prosthetic restoration that is too close to the alveolar bone crest

Crown lengthening can be limited to the soft tissues when there is enough gingiva coronal to the alveolar bone, allowing for surgical modification of the gingival margins without the need for osseous recontouring (i.e., pseudopockets in cases of gingival hyperplasia). An external or internal bevel gingivectomy (gingivoplasty) is the procedure of choice in these cases.

The biological width has not been compromised, and, as a result, the soft tissue pocket is eliminated and the teeth exposed without the need for osseous resection. Unfortunately, the majority of cases will involve bone recontouring as well as gingival resection to accommodate aesthetics and function. This is a more delicate procedure that requires exposing root surface, positioning gingival margins at the desired height, and apically reestablishing the biological width.

The crown-lengthening procedure enables restorative dentists to develop an adequate zone for crown retention without extending the crown margins deep into periodontal tissues. After the procedure, it is customary to wait 6–8 weeks before cementing the final restoration. In the aesthetic zone, a waiting period of at least 6 months is recommended before final impression (Pontoriero & Carnevale 2001). This reduces the chances of gingival recession following prosthetic crown insertion, specifically if there is a thin biotype.

A FEW WORDS ABOUT AESTHETICS

As the saying goes, "Beauty is in the eye of the beholder." Oral aesthetics is part art and part science. The enhancement of a person's smile culminates in the individualization of the general rules governing dental aesthetics for that person. Every patient is different, and yet a nice smile is the result of an orderly combination of several components. Knowing the general guidelines that make a smile appealing and tailoring them to an individual patient makes that smile unique.

The aesthetic zone has been defined as the area encompassed by the upper and lower lips (Saadoun & LeGall 1998). It is the harmonious relationship among the dentition (premolar to premolar), the periodontium (gingival line), and the lips that will make or break a smile.

Practical Periodontal Plastic Surgery, Second Edition. Edited by Serge Dibart.
© 2017 John Wiley & Sons, Inc. Published 2017 by John Wiley & Sons, Inc.

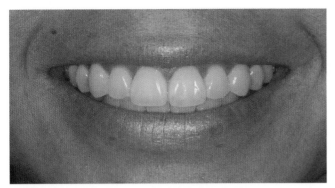

Figure 17.1 A pleasant smile line reveals 75–100% of the maxillary anterior teeth and the interproximal gingiva only (68.94% of the subjects). The gingival margins of the central incisors and canines are located horizontally at the same level, whereas the gingival margins of the laterals are 2 mm below. The maxillary incisal curve is parallel with the lower lip (84.8% of the subjects). Tjan et al. (1984). Reproduced with permission from Elsevier.

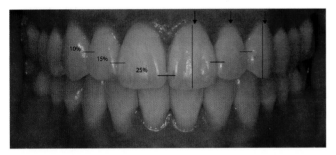

Figure 17.2 The position of the anterior contact point progressing from incisal to cervical and from central incisors to canines (*horizontal lines*). The location of the gingival zenith (*black arrows*), the most apical point of the gingival tissue, referencing the tooth axis, is distal on the maxillary central incisors and canines, and coincidental on lateral incisors (Rufenacht 2000). The *golden percentage* (25%, 15%, and 10%) is considered a starting point in designing the relative width of teeth in a beautiful smile. With all of these width ratios added together, the total canine-to-canine width becomes the *golden percentage*. Snow (1999). Reproduced with permission from Wiley.

In 1984, Tjan et al., after observing several hundred dental and hygiene students, defined a standard of normalcy in an aesthetic smile (Figs. 17.1 & 17.2).

ARMAMENTARIUM

This includes the basic kit plus crown-lengthening burrs and bone chisels.

SOFT TISSUE CROWN LENGTHENING

Soft tissue crown lengthening is best accomplished with an external or internal bevel gingivectomy. The alveolar bone is

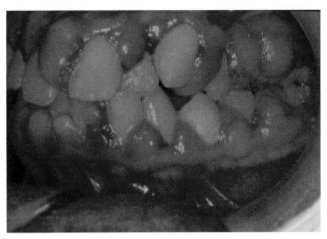

Figure 17.3 Gingival hyperplasia secondary to the daily use of Dilantin (phenytoin). This excessive tissue affects patients' dental aesthetics and function.

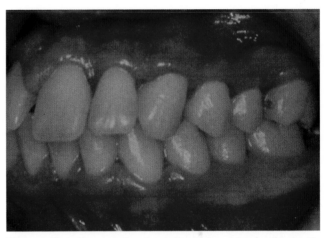

Figure 17.4 The mouth of a patient after minor orthodontic treatment and full-mouth external bevel gingivectomy. Hyperplastic gingival tissue has been surgically eliminated and the teeth exposed to the oral environment. As there is no need for osseous recontouring, the biological width is undisturbed.

left intact, the depth of the soft tissue pocket is marked with a probe (bleeding points) and a gingivectomy knife, Kirkland (Hu-Friedy, Chicago, IL, USA) or Orban (Hu-Friedy) (in case of external bevel gingivectomy), or a no. 15 blade (internal bevel gingivectomy) is used to eliminate that excess gingival (Figs. 17.3 and 17.4).

HARD TISSUE CROWN LENGTHENING

The optimal gingival line (margins) is determined after careful evaluation of the diagnostic waxup. A surgical guide is prepared from the waxup model that will help the surgeon re-create the ideal gingival line in the mouth. Using a no. 15 blade as a pencil, the surgeon outlines the incision and, following the surgical guide, keeps the blade at an angle to create a coronal internal bevel.

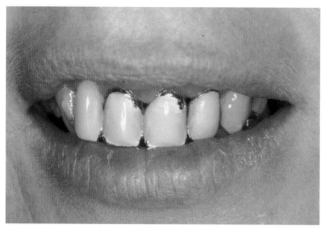

Figure 17.5 The mouth of a 42-year-old woman unhappy with her smile. Her lip line shows maxillary gingiva, iatrogenic dentistry, and erroneous gingival margin positions.

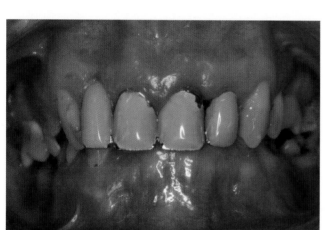

Figure 17.6 Intraoral photography shows a poorly designed prosthesis, severe overbite, faulty crown margins, and severely decayed teeth.

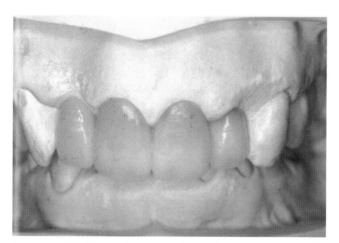

Figure 17.7 Diagnostic waxup from which a surgical guide will be created.

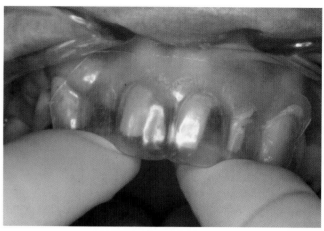

Figure 17.8 The provisional restorations are removed, and the surgical guide created from the waxup is inserted. This guides the surgeon to position the new gingival margins to the desired levels. The surgical incision follows the surgical guide closely to give the restorative dentist the precise amount of tooth structure needed to create a new gingival architecture.

The full-thickness flap is then reflected, the secondary flap discarded, and the bone exposed. Using burrs or bone chisels, the alveolar bone is recontoured to create a 3-mm space between the bone and the anticipated new margins. The flaps are sutured back in place and the area left to heal for about 3 weeks before repreparing the teeth (supragingivally) and relining the temporaries. A waiting period of about 6 months, in temporaries, is recommended in the aesthetic zone before final preparation and restoration (Figs. 17.5–17.14).

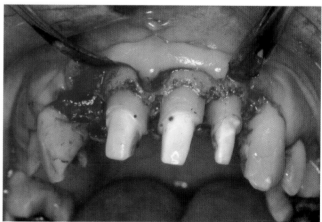

Figure 17.9 The full-thickness flap is elevated, and the osseous recontouring is done to expose the new tooth structure that will receive the new prosthetic margins. A 3-mm space between the bone crest and the planned new prosthetic margins is imperative for successful restoration.

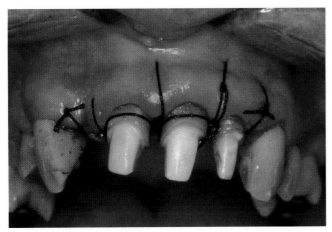

Figure 17.10 The flaps are secured with a continuous sling and vertical mattress suture.

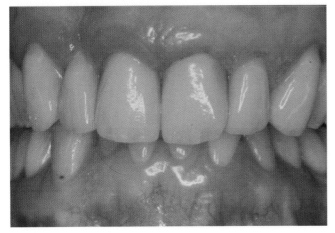

Figure 17.11 The final prosthesis is inserted 1 year later. The teeth have been customized to fit the patient's morphogenetic type.

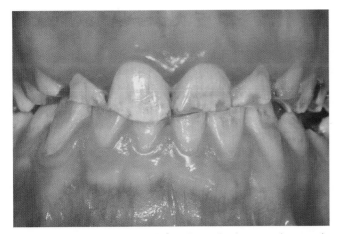

Figure 17.12 The mouth of a patient who has amelogenesis imperfecta. Extensive decay and short clinical crowns make it difficult for proper rehabilitation without crown lengthening.

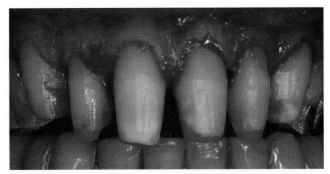

Figure 17.13 The surgical crown-lengthening procedure performed with removal of hard and soft tissues.

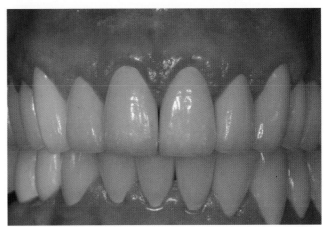

Figure 17.14 A patient's mouth rehabilitated aesthetically and functionally with individual porcelain fused to metal crowns.

MICROSURGICAL CROWN LENGTHENING

In the areas of high aesthetic demand, where papilla and soft tissue conservation is of paramount importance, the use of a microsurgical technique is recommended. There will be smaller incisions, which will not involve the papillae.

Flap reflection is minimal, and the sutures enable a very close adaptation of the flaps. This, in turn, results in minimal inflammation, scarring, and patient discomfort. Because of the minimally invasive nature of the procedures and the superior wound adaptation, quick healing and enhanced aesthetics are to be expected (Figs. 17.15–17.23).

MINIMALLY INVASIVE CROWN LENGTHENING WITH OR WITHOUT LIP REPOSITIONING

This technique is particularly useful in the anterior region when there is no need to reduce the bone levels interproximally. A surgical guide based on a diagnostic wax up can be used advantageously to determine the new gingival margins. A microsurgical scalpel is used to trim the excess gingiva and establish

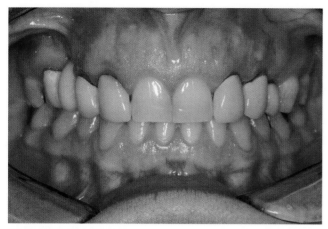

Figure 17.15 The mouth of a 40-year-old woman unhappy with her smile. She seeks help to improve her appearance and boost her self-confidence.

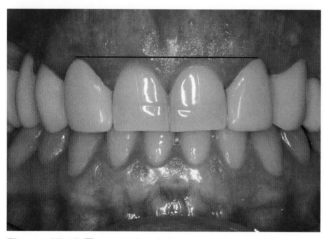

Figure 17.16 The mouth of the same patient after caries control and temporization. The condition has somewhat improved but notice the erroneous position of the gingival margins of teeth 8 and 9. They should be situated above the gingival margins of the lateral incisors.

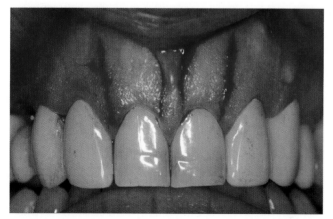

Figure 17.17 Two short vertical buccal incisions at the line angles of teeth 8 and 9 are made with a microblade leaving papillae and frenum intact. The mesial incisions are hidden in the labial frenum; this allows for invisible scarring.

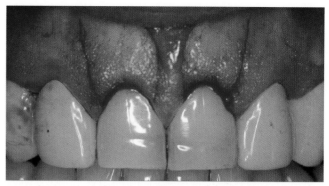

Figure 17.18 A submarginal incision mimicking the final gingival margin levels of teeth 8 and 9 will help connect the two verticals.

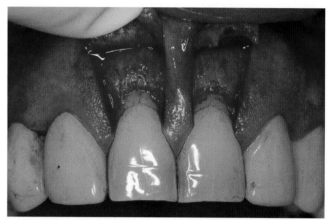

Figure 17.19 The full-thickness flaps are reflected just enough to expose crestal bone. The interdental papilla is left alone; this enhances a positive aesthetic outcome.

desired final gingival margins. Prior to the gingivectomy the supra osseous gingival unit needs to be recorded in order to accurately remove the alveolar bone and allow for the said unit to re-establish itself post surgically (Figs. 17.24 & 17.25). Failure to do so will result in the gingiva "bouncing back" (Scutella et al. 1999).

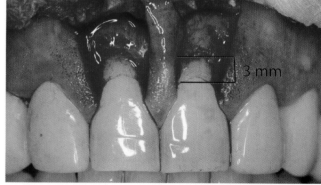

Figure 17.20 Crestal bone is removed with a chisel or a burr to have 3 mm of space between the anticipated prosthetic margins and the alveolar bone.

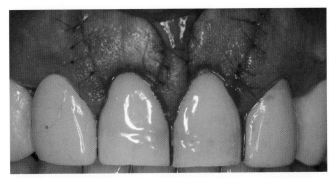

Figure 17.21 The flaps are sutured back in place with resorbable 7-0 microsutures. The number and position of the microsutures enable a close adaptation of the flaps and subsequent rapid healing.

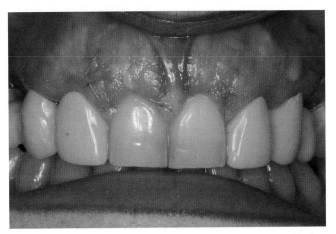

Figure 17.22 The mouth of the patient 1 week later. Notice the quality of the wound healing.

After the removal of the excised gingiva (Figs. 17.26 & 17.27), a small periosteal elevator (24G Hu Friedy) is used to delicately raise a full-thickness buccal flap without detaching the papillae. This is done in order to expose the underlying buccal alveolar bone that will be resected. The Piezotome (Satelec, Acteon-group) with the crown-lengthening insert CE3 is used to do the

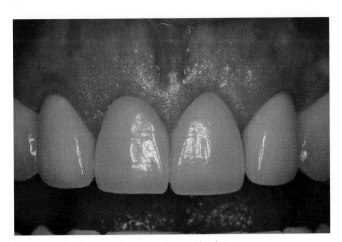

Figure 17.23 Final veneers 4 months later.

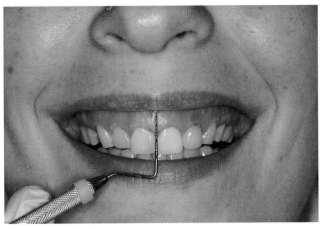

Figure 17.24 Patient complaining of a gummy smile. She is displaying excessive gingiva and has also upper lip hypermobility. The treatment plan for her will include crown lengthening and lip repositioning.

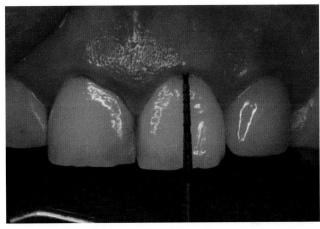

Figure 17.25 Subgingival insertion of the probe to record the length of the supraosseous gingival unit (tip of marginal gingiva to crest of alveolar bone).

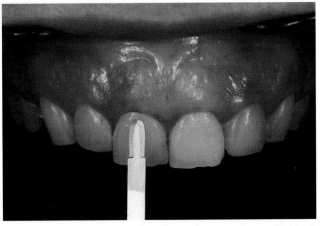

Figure 17.26 Using a microsurgical blade a submarginal incision will be made once local anesthesia is achieved.

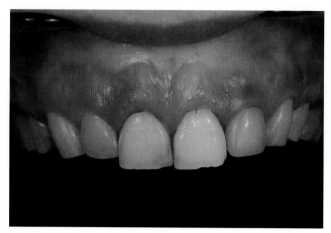

Figure 17.27 Submarginal incision and internal bevel gingivectomy has been done around the two central incisors.

ostectomy to the desired length. It is important not to damage the root surface during this procedure. A hand-operated mini bone chisel can be used to finish the ostectomy and do a small osteoplasty. The depth of the ostectomy is controlled with the periodontal probe to re-establish the natural gingival attachment unit (Figs. 17.28 & 17.29).

This unit has been measured and recorded at individual teeth buccal sites prior to the surgery and while the patient was anesthetized by inserting the periodontal probe into the sulcus and to the bone. This measure of the tooth's individual gingival attachment unit (from the free gingival margin to the tip of the alveolar bone) will have to be duplicated scrupulously to avoid the gingiva "bouncing back" post surgery.

Once this gingival attachment unit space has been reestablished apically, the gingiva is "pressed" back on the teeth/bone using a wet gauze and fingers for 2–3 min. Postsurgical healing is usually uneventful and rapid (Fig. 17.30).

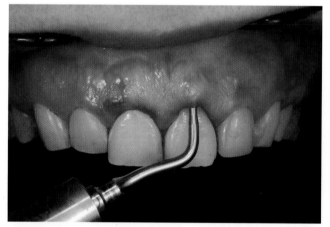

Figure 17.28 The gingiva is lifted away from the underlying bone gently using a microsurgical periosteal elevator. The piezotome with the crown-lengthening tip is inserted under the gingiva and used to do the ostectomy.

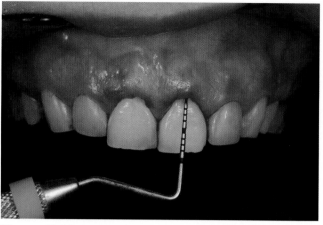

Figure 17.29 A probe is inserted subgingivally to measure the distance between the tip of the gingiva and the alveolar bone, making sure to duplicate the original distance of the supraosseous gingival unit. Removing the correct amount of bone will help re-establish the space needed for the supraosseous gingival unit.

The patient is back a month later to proceed with the lip repositioning procedure (Rosenblatt & Simon 2006; Simon et al. 2007). After local anesthesia, the area to be operated is marked with an indelible pencil. Using a scalpel with a no. 15 blade the sharp dissection is carried out to remove the superficial mucosal layer of the inner lip. A scissor can also be used to help with the dissection. Lip-lifting muscles should not be severed during this procedure. Once the dissection is finished, the two edges of the mucosa are sutured back together using single interrupted sutures. These sutures would have to stay for 6–8 weeks (Figs. 17.31–17.35).

The patient is then discharged with postoperative instructions.

It is important to emphasize to the patient the possibility of some degree of relapse in the future (Figs. 17.36 & 17.37).

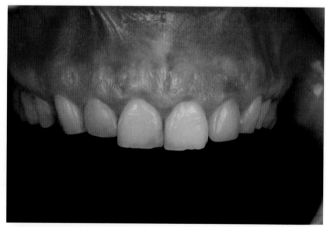

Figure 17.30 The patient 2 weeks post crown-lengthening surgery on teeth 8 and 9.

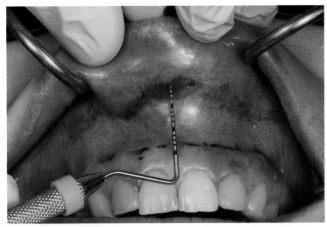

Figure 17.31 The patient 1 month later. The amount of mucosa to be removed has been determined and the surgical area mapped using a blue pencil.

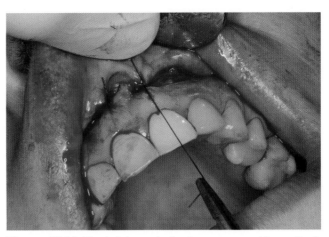

Figure 17.34 Single interrupted sutures are used to reattach the mucosal edges.

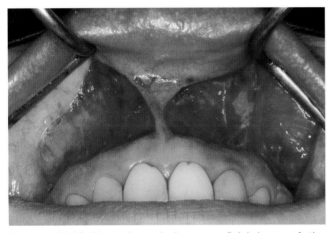

Figure 17.32 Dissection of the superficial layer of the mucosa using a scalpel with a no. 15 blade and scissors. The maxillary frenum is left in place to facilitate accurate repositioning of the lip.

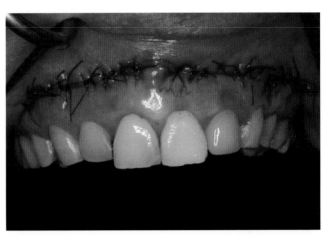

Figure 17.35 The area sutured. These sutures will stay in for 6–8 weeks.

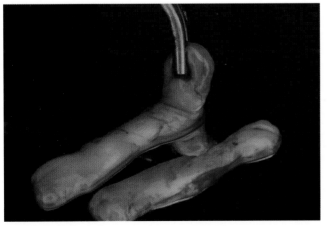

Figure 17.33 The mucosal tissue excised.

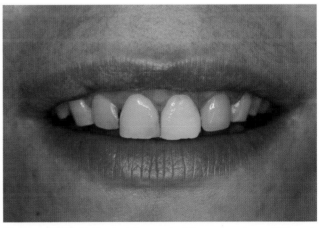

Figure 17.36 Patient at the end of the procedure. Although the result is very satisfactory, the patient should be told of the possibility of some relapse in the coming years. Image courtesy of Dr. Eihab Mously.

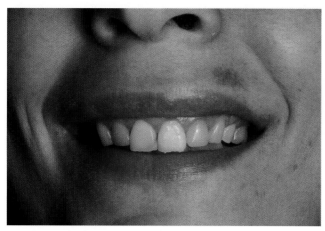

Figure 17.37 Patient 2 weeks post surgery. Courtesy Dr. Eihab Mously.

REFERENCES

Cohen, D.W. (1962) Periodontal preparation of the mouth for restorative dentistry. Presented at the Walter Reed Army Medical Center, Washington, DC, 3 June 1962.

de Waal, H., & Castellucci, G. (1994) The importance of restorative margin placement to the biologic width and periodontal health. Part II. *International Journal of Periodontics and Restorative Dentistry* 14, 70–83.

Gargiulo, A.W., Wentz, F.M., & Orban, B. (1961) Dimensions and relations of the dentogingival junction in humans. *Journal of Periodontology* 32, 261–267.

Ingber, J.S. (1976) Forced eruption. Part II. A method of treating non-restorable teeth: Periodontal and restorative considerations. *Journal of Periodontology* 47, 203–213.

Ingber, F.J.S., Rose, L.F., & Coslet, J.G. (1977) The biologic width: A concept in periodontics and restorative dentistry. *Alpha Omegan* 10, 62–65.

Parma-Benfenati, S., Fugazzotto, P.A., & Ruben, M.P. (1985) The effect of restorative margins on the post-surgical development and nature of the periodontium. Part I. *International Journal of Periodontics and Restorative Dentistry* 5(6), 30–51.

Pontoriero, R., & Carnevale, G. (2001) Surgical crown lengthening: A 12-month clinical wound healing study. *Journal of Periodontology* 72, 841–848.

Pontoriero, R., Celenza, F., Jr., Ricci, G., & Carnevale, M. (1987) Rapid extrusion with fiber resection: A combined orthodontic-periodontic treatment modality. *International Journal of Periodontics and Restorative Dentistry* 5, 30–43.

Rosenblatt, A., & Simon, Z. (2006) Lip repositioning for reduction of excessive gingival display: A clinical report. *International Journal of Periodontics and Restorative Dentistry* 26, 433–437.

Rufenacht, C.R. (2000) *Principles of Esthetic Integration. London: Quintessence*, 13–36.

Saadoun, A.P., & LeGall, M.G. (1998) Periodontal implications in implant treatment planning for aesthetic results. *Practical Periodontics and Aesthetic Dentistry* 10, 655–664.

Scutella, F., Landi, L., Stellino, G., & Morgano, S.M. (1999) Surgical template for crown lengthening: A clinical report. *Journal of Prosthetic Dentistry* 82(3), 253–256.

Simon, Z., Rosemblatt, A., & Dorfmann, W. (2007) Eliminating a gummy smile with surgical lip repositioning. *Journal of Cosmetic Dentistry* 23, 100–108.

Snow, S.R. (1999) Esthetic smile analysis of maxillary anterior tooth width: The golden percentage. *Journal of Esthetic Dentistry* 11, 177–184.

Tal, H., Soldinger, M., Dreiangel, A., & Pitaru, S. (1989) Periodontal response to long-term abuse of the gingival attachment by supracrestal amalgam restorations. *Journal of Clinical Periodontology* 16, 654–689.

Tarnow, D., Sthal, S.S., Magner, A., & Zamzok, J. (1986) Human gingival attachment responses to subgingival crown placement–marginal remodeling. *Journal of Clinical Periodontology* 13, 563–569.

Tjan, A.H., Miller, G.D., & The, J.G. (1984) Some esthetic factors in a smile. *Journal of Prosthetic Dentistry* 51, 24–28.

Chapter 18 Introduction to Minimally Invasive Facial Aesthetic Procedures

Bradford Towne

OVERVIEW

Today, neurotoxins and temporary facial fillers are the top cosmetic procedures purchased by the public, replacing more invasive procedures such as face lifts and facial peels. According to a 12-year retrospective analysis conducted by the American Society of Plastic Surgeons, major facial cosmetic procedures declined by 27% in one 3-year period (2006–2009) (Remington 2008), while minimally invasive procedures (MIP) increased during the 12-year study period. Neurotoxin use increased by 680% and soft tissue fillers increased by 205% during the same period (Sandoval et al. 2014). Facial fillers have been available for decades but only in the last dozen years has there been the development of fillers that are technically easy to use, non-allergenic, give predictable results, are easily manipulated and sculpted by the injector, and have minimal risk of complications. Neurotoxins have also been available for years. They were first isolated and potential medical uses described in 1822. The source of the toxin, however, was not isolated until 80 years later (Foster 2014). Neurotoxins for cosmetic use were first approved by the US Food and Drink Administration (FDA) in 2002. Since then they have become the most commonly used cosmetic procedure by far, with soft tissue facial fillers the second most common cosmetic procedure performed.

The clinician that provides his or her patients with cosmetic neurotoxins and soft tissue fillers must have a detailed understanding of facial anatomy and the mechanics of the muscles of facial expression. A thorough appreciation of the aging process, including the physiologic changes that occur to skin, subcutaneous tissues, and muscles of the face, is critical to successfully treating cosmetic patients. This knowledge must be combined with an in-depth understanding of the pharmacology and working properties of the products to be used to restore facial volume. The clinician must also have an appreciation for the artistic qualities of the human facial form to be successful in creating an aesthetically pleasing result for the patient.

PATIENT SELECTION AND ASSESSMENT

Patient motivation for seeking MIPs varies tremendously but can be divided into three primary sectors. Young patients, generally 18–35, are usually motivated by the desire to augment an area of their face they feel is deficient or not normal. Those in the 35–55 age group are usually seeking rejuvenation and the 55+ are usually looking for restoration. All are looking for MIPs with minimal downtime, providing minimal risks and rapid results.

MIPs are generally procedures with minimal risks and complications when performed correctly and on the right patients. Fortunately, there are few medical contraindications for the use of neurotoxins or facial fillers today. Success in providing MIPs is the result of a careful evaluation of the patient's motivation in seeking treatment as well as a complete facial assessment. Cosmetic patients may have unrealistic expectations of what can be accomplished with MIPs and the clinician must be able educate the patient about realistic outcomes.

The evaluation begins with the patient describing what they are unhappy with about their face. This provides a starting point for the examination. It provides the clinician with an initial focal point to understand a patient's motivation. For example, a patient may tell the clinician that family and friends tell them they always look angry or tired. A patient may say that their cheeks look flat or hollow. Some patients describe the loss of lip exposure. Each of these complaints provides a starting point for the clinical evaluation. Once the patient's primary concern/complaint and treatment goal is ascertained the clinician can perform a comprehensive facial evaluation and develop treatment recommendations to achieve the patient's goal.

No evaluation is complete without a review of the patient's past medical history, medications, and social history, including sun exposure, smoking and history of any prior facial cosmetic procedures. The examination should include an assessment

Practical Periodontal Plastic Surgery, Second Edition. Edited by Serge Dibart.
© 2017 John Wiley & Sons, Inc. Published 2017 by John Wiley & Sons, Inc.

Table 18.1 Glogau Classification of Photo Aging and Wrinkles

Group	Classification	Typical Age	Description	Skin Characteristics
I	Mild	28–35	No wrinkles	Early photo aging: mild pigment changes, no keratosis, minimal wrinkles, minimal or no make-up
II	Moderate	35–50	Wrinkles in motion (dynamic rhytids)	Early to moderate photo aging: early brown spots visible, keratosis palpable but not visible, parallel smile lines begin to appear, wears some foundation
III	Advanced	50–65	Wrinkles at rest (static rhytids)	Advanced photo aging: obvious discolorations, visible capillaries (telangiectasia), visible keratosis, wears heavier foundation always
IV	Severe	60–75	Only wrinkles	Severe photo aging: yellow–gray skin color, prior skin malignancies, wrinkles throughout, no normal skin, cannot wear make-up because it cakes and cracks

of the skin condition using the Glogau Classification of Photo Aging and Wrinkles (Table 18.1).

The physical evaluation should follow the three facial esthetic zones as first described by Leonardo da Vinci. These three zones divide the face horizontally into thirds. The top extends from the top of the forehead to the inferior orbital rim. The midface extends from the inferior orbital rim to the base of the nose. The lower third extends from the nasal base to the chin.

It is useful in this evaluation to have a frontal facial diagram on which the clinician can indicate the location of static and dynamic wrinkles, areas of volume loss, redundant or sagging skin, and deep folds. Consent should be obtained and pre-treatment photos and or videos obtained to demonstrate the areas of concern. Videos are particularly useful in demonstrating dynamic vs static rhytids. Preexisting facial asymmetries should also be noted. This is very important to document so that the patient is made aware of their existence prior to any treatment administration. Once the evaluation is complete, the clinical findings should be reviewed with the patient and treatment recommendations discussed in detail, including the rationale, expected result, and potential risks and complications. If different products are available to treat the same problem, the benefits and risks of each should be reviewed.

NEUROTOXINS

Currently there are three neurotoxin products available for cosmetic uses: Botox Cosmetic®, Dysport® and Xeomin®. All of these are derivatives of BoNT A. Use of botulinum toxin type A (BoNT A) derivatives is FDA approved to treat glabellar frown lines. Botox Cosmetic® has been approved for crow's feet treatment. Each derivative has its own specific unit concentration but the results are similar (Rubin 2013).

Common adverse effects at the injection site include pain, bruising, erythema, and edema. The most common general adverse effects are headaches, upper respiratory tract infections, nausea, pain, and flu-like symptoms.

TEMPORARY AND SEMI-PERMANENT FILLERS

The first cosmetic filler used was paraffin in 1899 (Kontis & Rivkin 2009). Its popularity was short lived as the complications associated with its use quickly exceeded the benefits. Today, there are many types of temporary and semi-permanent facial fillers available on the market. The most commonly utilized are the hyaluronic acid (HA) fillers. These fillers (Restylane®/Perlane®, Juvaderm®and Belotero®) are composed of micro particles of hyaluronic acid, a naturally occurring substance in our body with the highest concentrations found in the connective tissue and fluid around our eyes and also in some cartilage and joint fluid. HA fillers are synthetically derived and are more concentrated than those naturally found in our bodies. The injected gel provides a volume greater than the volume injected because it is hydrophilic (draws water into the area of injection). It is important not to over-inject because of this delayed phenomenon. The material is slowly degraded over time. The microspheres vary in size by product and the indications for the use of each are based on the desired effect. The small particle sizes are used for wrinkle ablation and the larger sizes for volume replacement.

Another commonly utilized product is hydroxyapatite filler (Radiesse®). This product is composed of microspheres of hydroxyapatite crystal (a component of bone) suspended in a gel matrix. The mechanism of action is immediate volume enhancement (what you see is what you get). Over time the degradation of the hydroxyapatite stimulates collagenesis. Although this new collagen is not permanent it does prolong the benefit of the treatment.

Neither hyaluronic acid nor hydroxyapatite produces an allergic response or requires allergy testing. Most HA products provide 12–18 months of benefit. Hydroxyapatite gel will usually provide 18–24 months of volume enhancement. Both product types are relatively risk free with minimal complications such as bruising (Table 18.2). An important distinction between the two is the reversibility of HA by injecting the treated area with hyaluronidase.

Table 18.2 Properties of hyaluronic acid fillers and hydroxyapatite filler

Hyaluronic acid fillers (Restylane®/Perlane®, Juvaderm® and Belotero®)
Lasts 6–12 months (Juvaderm Voluma 18–24 months)
Maximum volume effect takes several days due to hydrophilic volume
Identical in all species and tissues
Isovolemic degradation
No skin test required
Reversible
Hydroxyapatite filler (Radiesse®)
Lasts 12–18 months
Provides an immediate volumizing effect
Stimulates the patient's own collagen to produce a satisfying and longer lasting result
Less volume required per equivalent treatment compared to HA fillers to achieve the same result

TREATMENT SEQUENCING

Treatment sequencing is based on the products to be used and the areas to be treated. Generally, treatment should begin with neurotoxins followed by facial fillers. If both are to be injected into the same area it is best to wait a week after administration of the neurotoxin prior to injecting the fillers. Injecting filler into the area of a hyperkinetic muscle will likely result in the displacement of the filler away from the intended site. Facial fillers placed in the midface to increase volume will elevate the nasolabial folds and lower face. This effect will result in less volume replacement being required when treating the lower face.

Fig. 18.1 (which is available from Allergan for providers enrolled in their website) is a useful teaching and treatment planning tool. The clinician can show the patient the areas to be treated and draw out the treatment solution being recommended. The individual muscles to be treated with neurotoxin can be identified along with the injection sites. For fillers, the area to be treated can be highlighted along with the planned injection patterns.

NEUROTOXIN INJECTION TECHNIQUE

The neurotoxin of choice should be reconstituted following the package insert guidelines. Typically injections are done with a TB or insulin syringe with a 30- or 32-gauge needle. The neurotoxin is measured in units. Vials come in either 50-unit or 100-unit doses. Individual injections sites usually have between 2 and 10 units depending on the product being used. Insertion of the needle is just into the body of the muscle being treated except when treating crow's feet, when the injection should be subcutaneous due to the orbicularis oculi muscle being very thin and superficial laterally. The most common area of treatment is the vertical glabellae rhytids. These furrows form as the result of the activity of the procerus and corrugator muscles, which pull the lower middle forehead down and toward the center, creating single, double or triple furrows (also known as the 1s, 11s, and 111s). The crow's feet formed as the result of the contraction of the lateral aspect of the orbicularis oculi is

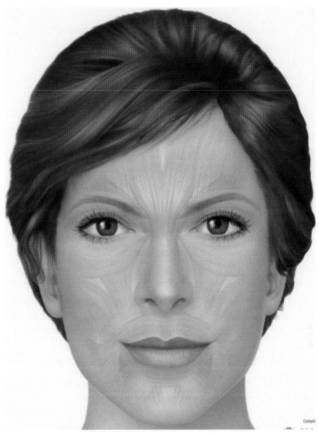

Figure 18.1 Subcutaneous facial muscles (available from Allergan for providers enrolled in their website). Adapted from botoxcosmetic.com.

the second most common area of neurotoxin treatment, followed by the forehead.

The glabellar (11s) lines arise from the action of the procerus and corrugator supercilii muscles (Figs. 18.2 & 18.3). These muscles tend to be hyperdynamic and when coupled with loss of subcutaneous fat and repetitive creasing result in the development of static wrinkles and potential textural changes. The lines usually appear between the muscle bodies as the subcutaneous fat volume shrinks.

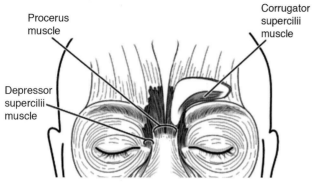

Figure 18.2 The glabellar muscle complex that creates the frown lines.

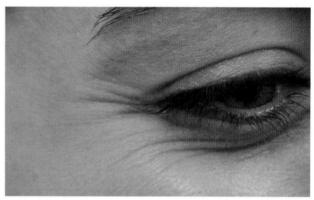

Figure 18.4 Hyperdynamic orbicularis oculi resulting in crow's feet rhytids.

Crow's feet or smile lines (Fig. 18.4) are the result of the activity of the lateral aspect of the orbicularis oculi. The muscle's hyperdynamic activity combined with subcutaneous fat loss and repetitive creasing produce textural and static wrinkles lateral to the eye.

Forehead wrinkles (Fig. 18.5) are the result of the action of frontalis muscle. They produce horizontal wrinkles. The wrinkles become deeper and more exaggerated as the result of the loss of subcutaneous fat, photoaging, and loss of dermal elasticity. Repetitive creasing also produces textural changes to the epidermis.

Neurotoxins are measured in units, for example Botox Cosmetic® and Xeomin® come in either 100-unit or 50-unit vials. The recommended reconstitution of a 100-unit vial of Botox Cosmetic® requires the addition of 2.5 cc of non-preserved sterile saline for injection. This volume yields a concentration of 40 units per 1 cc or 4 units per 0.1 cc. A typical number of units of Botox Cosmetic® recommended for a glabellar injection site is 4 units or 0.1 cc. Use of 1-cc TB syringes or 1-cc insulin syringes is necessary to deliver accurate volume and concentration of the neurotoxin to the sites (Fig. 18.6). This volume will produce a small wheel, minimize discomfort, and limit the diffusion radius to about 1 cm. The dose for each site is individualized based on the examination, including the muscle thickness, degree of hyperkinetic activity,

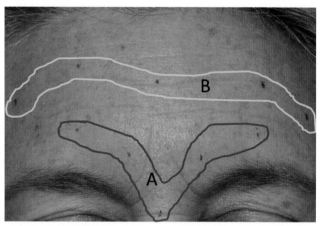

Figure 18.5 Glabellar frown rhytids (A) and horizontal forehead rhytids (B) (the result of frontalis action) with marks indicating planned injection sites of neurotoxin

and past patient results. Each product has different suggested dilutent instructions and the clinician should refer to the package insert of each product for those instructions.

When injecting the frown lines (glabellar) there are typically five injection sites that correspond to the bodies of the procerus and corrugator muscles. Fig. 18.7 demonstrates the usual locations of these injection sites. It is important to stay 1 cm

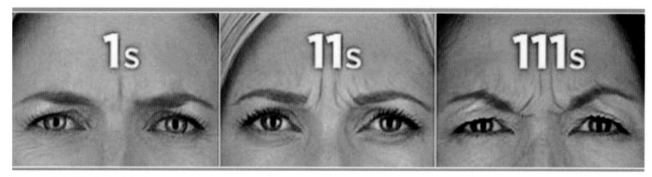

Figure 18.3 Vertical glabellae rhytids: single, double andr triple furrows (also known as the 1s, 11s, and 111s). Adapted from botoxcosmetic.com.

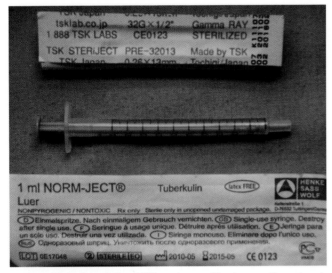

Figure 18.6 Specialized TB syringe with plunger tip extending into hub to reduce waste with each syringe, coupled with a 32-gauge needle to minimize the discomfort of injections.

above the superior orbital rim to avoid diffusion of the product into the upper eyelid. The eyebrow position is a poor landmark to use due to its variable location. The boney orbital rim should always be palpated and the injection given 1 cm above this landmark. The action of the corrugator muscle should be observed as its location may be more vertical in some individuals. Fig. 18.8 shows the typical lateral injection site at mid-pupil, with the patient looking straight ahead. Each injection is typically 2–4 units of Botox Cosmetic® or Xeomin® or 5–10 units of Dysport®.

The forehead horizontal lines (Fig. 18.9) can also be treated but caution should be observed if injecting at the same time as the glabellar frown lines. If complete frontalis paralysis occurs the patient may present with eyebrow ptosis. A couple of centimeters of frontalis should be kept inferiorly untreated to insure that this does not happen.

Crow's feet or smile lines (Fig. 18.10) are easily treated at the same time as the glabellar lines. By reducing hyperdynamic activity before static creases develop the occurrence of static wrinkles can be postponed. Care should be taken not to extend

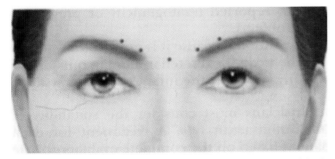

Figure 18.7 Typical injection sites for treatment of the glabellar lines. Adapted from xeominaesthetic.com.

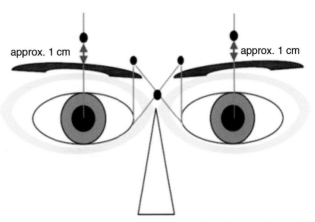

Figure 18.8 The location of each injection site relative to the eyes. Adapted from xeominaesthetic.com.

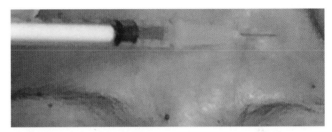

Figure 18.9 Injection of the left lateral site (corrugator muscle).

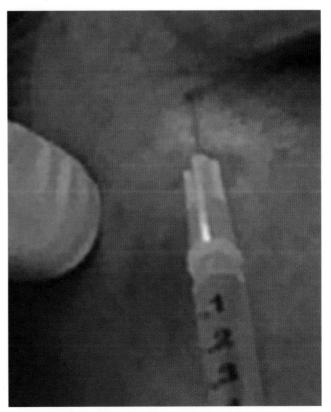

Figure 18.10 Injection of the orbicularis oculi 1 cm lateral to the orbital rim at the mid-canthus level. It is important to remain quite superficial in this area.

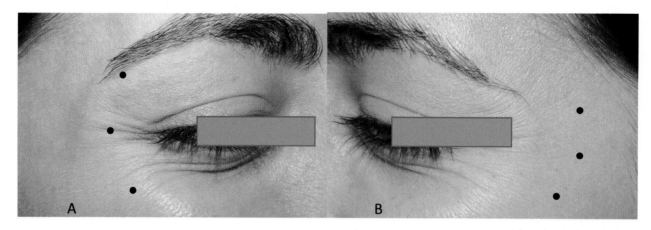

Before

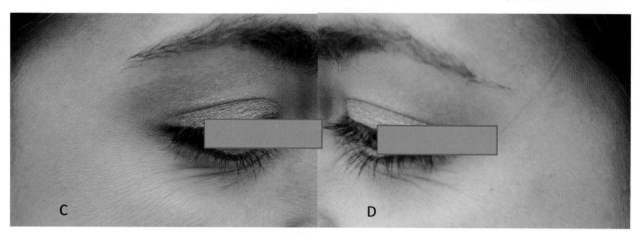

1 week after injection

Figure 18.11 Top: 1 week post injection results of neurotoxin ablation of crow's feet showing the left (A) and right (B) preinjections. Bottom: 1 week post injection, left (C) and right (D).

the injections into the inferior orbital rim area as this increases the risk of producing a result that looks like a mask, with no animation at all when smiling. Crow's feet are usually treated with a dose of 2 units of Botox Cosmetic® or Xeomin® or 5 units of Dysport® per injection site. The injection of the crow's feet is just subcutaneous due to the superficial position of the orbicularis oculi laterally. Caution should be exercised as there are superficial veins in this area that must be avoided. These veins are often visible when the skin is stretched during the injections. The superior injection is usually at the lateral aspect of the eyebrow, the next is level with the canthus, and the lower is inferiolateral. Each should be 1 cm from the bony orbital rim (Fig. 18.11).

TREATMENT OF THE MIDFACE AND LOWER FACE WITH FILLERS

Volume loss plays a much more important role in aging in the mid and lower face than hyperdynamic muscle activity. When

evaluating the midface the fullness of the cheeks should be assessed even though this is not usually an area the patient is aware of. Cheek volume can profoundly affect the appearance of the nasolabial folds, marionette lines, and prejowl sulcus. Deep folds such as the nasolabial and marionette lines are the result of loss of subcutaneous fat from the height of the cheek bones to the inferior border of the mandible. This loss of fat results in skin sags and laxity, creating a tired and older looking face. The combination of this with the loss of the structural framework to support the skin (collagen and elastin) and surface wrinkles further complicates the aging process.

Lip volume is an important visual component of the face. Lips, particularly in women, play a major role in defining beauty and youthfulness in most cultures. An upper lip that is a flat, poorly defined white roll with narrowing of the Cupid's bow and lack of fullness of the vermillion border is generally considered deficient and lacking in beauty. Add to this the vertical rhytids associated with aging, volume loss, smoking, and photoaging

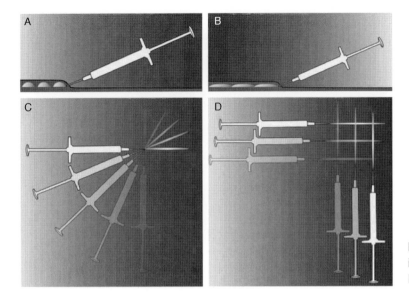

Figure 18.12 (A) Serial puncture, (B) linear threading, (C) fanning, and (D) cross-hatching. From Rohrich et al. (2007).

and you have a very old looking first impression of the face. Neurotoxins cannot address these deficiencies. Augmentations with some form of filler or implants are the only viable solution for treating these volume deficiencies. Even full or modified facelifts ultimately only remove redundant skin and tighten the skin over a volume-deficient face.

The temporary and semi-permanent fillers available offer a patient treatment options with reduced risks and complications compared to the fillers available previously, but they yield similar longevity and offer patients minimal down-time for "recovery". For the clinician, the fillers are easy to use and offer predictable results when properly administered, and one class of fillers (HA) are reversible.

Injection techniques are varied and are dependent on both the location of injection and clinician preference. Typical techniques (Fig. 18.12) include linear threading, fanning, cross-hatching, and serial puncture.

When using HA for fine wrinkle ablation a linear threading technique usually works best. Injection on withdrawal in usually easier and more comfortable for the patient but there is

slightly higher risk of bruising as the needle is pushed forward intradermally. Injection on advancement offers the benefit of a reduced risk of bruising because filler is injected ahead of the needle, opening up a space.

For volume enhancement, several techniques are available. Cross-hatching works particularly well for marionette lines and the mouth corners as well as in the area below the zygoma and zygomatic arch. For the nasolabial folds, midface/cheekbones, and pre-jowl sulcus deep linear threading or fanning tends to work best. Alternatively, there are clinicians who prefer to inject small intermittent aliquots of filler then massage and shape the product into the area they desire to enhance. Most fillers need to be gently massaged and shaped after placement. This is where an understanding of what constitutes beauty and ideal facial form is critical.

Many patients arrive with a primary complaint of deep nasolabial folds and a flat thin upper lip. Often, in spite of other areas of volume deficits, these are the key areas of concern. The next areas of concern are the marionette lines and pre-jowl sulcus. These areas are usually easy to evaluate for the clinician and injection techniques are straightforward (Fig. 18.13).

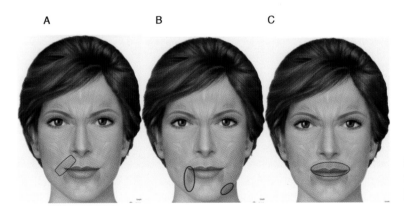

Figure 18.13 (A) Nasolabial folds injection site, (B) marionette lines and pre jowl sulcus, and (C) upper lip.

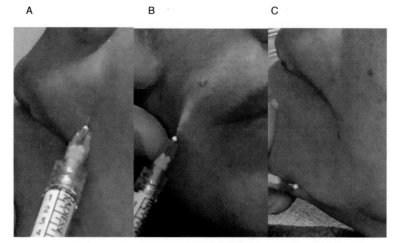

Figure 18.14 Linear injection on withdrawal technique used in the placement of Radiesse® at the subdermal/dermal junction to provide fill and ablation of (A) nasolabial fold, (B) junction nasolabial fold and marionette line, and (C) prejowl sulcus.

In evaluating the nasolabial folds, look at how deep they are. Are the folds narrow or wide? Do they sag over the upper lip? Is there any hyperdynamic activity resulting in the upper lip folding under the midface? Is there any asymmetry? Is the lip flat with vertical rhytids? Is there a white roll? Is the columella well defined or flat? Are there any vertical folds at the corners of the mouth extending toward the inferior border of the mandible? Does the inferior border of the mandible in front of the masseter muscle insertion show a depression?

Once the injection sites have been identified, the product to be used must be selected. HA fillers come in various particle sizes and are available from multiple companies. For fine wrinkles and shallow (intradermal) injections, HA products are always the best choice. Deep volume enhancement can be accomplished with either HA products or the hydroxyapatite product, Radiesse® (Fig. 18.14).

The volume of product injected will vary by site and the degree of deficit to be filled. In most cases to treat a patient with moderate nasolabial folds will take at least two 1 cc syringes of HA product or 1.8 cc of Radiesse® (Fig. 18.15). There is always a delicate balance of overtreatment vs under treatment. It is always better to undertreat and tell the patient that a reassessment will be done in 7–10 days and touch up carried out as needed as opposed to a patient returning complaining of excessive fill. Although HA products are reversible with hyaluronidase, the result is usually the loss of the entire product. Radiesse®, on the other hand, is not reversible. It can be manipulated up to 7 days post injection by warming with moist heat packs and then massaging, which can disperse some overfill but not eliminate it.

Lip augmentation consists of two components. Definition of the vermillion border by re-establishing the white roll plays a major role in revitalizing the lips. This interrupts fine vertical rhytids from continuing from the skin onto the mucosa and creates a distinct light reflection at the junction of the mucosa and the skin of each lip. In some lips where volume has significantly diminished or in the edentulous patient with a combination of alveolar atrophy and lip sagging, volume enhancement may be appropriate. In the upper lip this is accomplished with the placement of pillows of filler in the body of the lip where the arch of the upper lip is highest bilaterally. The lower lip is augmented with a pillow placed in the body at the mid third of the lip (Fig. 18.16).

MIPs such as neurotoxins, and temporary and semi-permanent facial fillers offer patients the opportunity enhance and restore

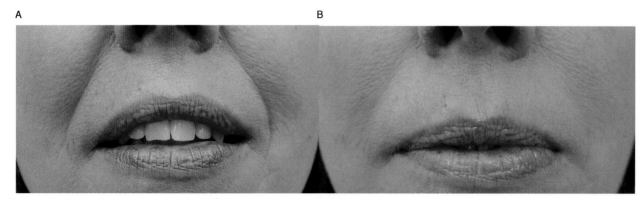

Figure 18.15 A 1.8-ml syringe Radiesse® filler was used to fill the nasolabial folds: (A) pre injection, (B) 1 week post injection. Linear threading and fanning on withdrawal were used to achieve the final result.

A   B

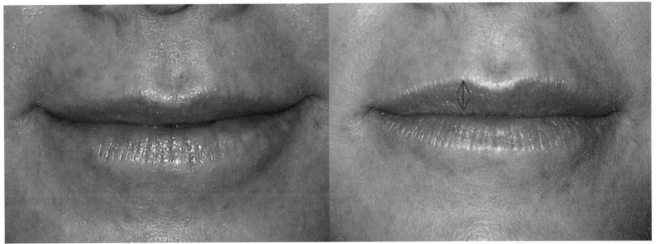

Figure 18.16 (A) Pre injection with topical anesthetic cream on lips (note the reversed ratio of upper lip to lower lip here) and (B) 2 months post injection. Notice the improved definition of the white roll (the junction between the mucosa and the skin). The increased height of the upper lip creates a more balanced relationship with the lower lip. The Cupid's bow has better projection and fullness.

not only their oral cavity but also the extra-oral facial appearance, allowing a complete facial makeover without undergoing more invasive procedures requiring extensive recovery time. The key motivators for patients seeking aesthetic procedures fall into roughly three categories: augmentation, rejuvenation, and restoration. These vary in the population primarily based on the age range of the individual. Youth seeks augmentation, looking for improvement over what they have, middle age (post children) generally are looking to rejuvenate and bring back what has declined over time, and the seniors are looking for the restoration of what has been lost. Awareness of these generational motivators helps clinicians identify what the treatment goals are for their patient. This then helps to customize the treatment plan to reach the patient's objectives. The difficulty is making sure that a patient's desired outcome is achievable and not unrealistic. Treatment should be directed to match the generational timeline. You cannot not esthetically take a senior and enhance them in the same way as you would a youthful patient.

REFERENCES

Foster, K.A. (2014) Molecular Aspects of Botulinum Neurotoxin. In: *Overview and History of Botulinum Toxin Research, Current Topics in Neurotoxicity*, pp. 1–7. Springer.

Kontis, T., & Rivkin, A. (2009) The history of injectable facial fillers. *Facial Plastic Surgery* 25(2), 67–71.

Remington, B.K. (2008) Facial contouring and volumization. Medscape Dermatology, Remington Laser Centre, Calgary.

Rohrich, R.J., Ghavami, A., & Crosby, M.A. (2007) The role of hyaluronic acid fillers (restylane) in facial cosmetic surgery: review and technical considerations. *Plastic Reconstructive Surgery* 120(6 Suppl), 41S–54S.

Rubin, M. (2013) Neurotoxins: Clinical perspective on subtle differences. *Practical Dermatology* January, 29–32.

Sandoval, L., Huang, K., Davis, S., Feldman, S., & Taylor, S. (2014) Trends in the use of neurotoxins and dermal fillers by US physicians. *Journal of Clinical and Aesthetic Dermatology* 7(9), 14–19.

Chapter 19 Selection Criteria

Serge Dibart and Mamdouh Karima

The proper selection of numerous techniques must be based on the predictability of success that, in turn, is based on the criteria discussed in this chapter.

PLAQUE-FREE AND INFLAMMATION-FREE ENVIRONMENT

Periodontal plastic surgical procedures should be performed in a plaque-free and inflammation-free environment to enable firm gingival tissue management. When the tissue is inflamed and edematous, precise incision lines and flap reflection cannot be achieved. The patient's teeth must undergo careful and thorough scaling, root planning, and meticulous plaque control before any surgical procedure.

AESTHETIC DEMAND

Short-term clinical studies show that the connective tissue graft results in superior root coverage compared with the epithelialized free soft tissue graft. In addition, the color match of the grafted area to the adjacent gingiva is aesthetically more favorable with the connective tissue graft than with an epithelialized free graft.

ADEQUATE BLOOD SUPPLY

Maximum blood supply to the donor tissue is essential. Gingival augmentation apical to the area of recession benefits from a better blood supply than coronal augmentation because the recipient bed is entirely vascular (periosteum). Root-coverage procedures are a challenge because a portion of the bed is avascular (the portion of the root to be covered). Therefore, if aesthetics is not a factor, gingival augmentation apical to the recession may have a more predictable outcome.

A pedicle-displaced flap has a better blood supply than a free graft (since the base of the flap is intact in the former). Therefore, in root coverage, if the anatomy is favorable, the use of a pedicle flap or any of its variants may be the best procedure.

The pouch and tunnel techniques use a split flap for a subepithelial connective tissue graft, with the connective tissue sandwiched in between the flap. This flap design maximizes the blood supply to the donor tissue. If large areas require root coverage, these sandwich-type recipient sites provide the best flap design for blood supply.

ANATOMY OF THE RECIPIENT AND DONOR SITES

The anatomy of the recipient and donor sites is an important consideration in selecting the proper technique. The presence or absence of vestibular depth is an essential anatomical criterion at the recipient site for gingival augmentation. If gingival augmentation is indicated apical to the area of recession, there must be adequate vestibular depth apical to the recessed gingival margin to provide space for either a free or pedicle graft.

Only a free graft can accomplish vestibular depth apical to the recession. Mucogingival techniques, such as free gingival grafts and free connective tissue grafts, should be used to create vestibular depth and widen the zone of attached gingiva. Other techniques require the presence of the vestibule before the surgery. These procedures include pedicle grafts (lateral and coronal), subepithelial connective tissue grafts, and pouch and tunnel procedures.

DONOR TISSUE AVAILABILITY

Pedicle displacement of tissue necessitates the creation of an adjacent donor site presenting the appropriate gingival thickness and width. Palatal tissue thickness is necessary for the connective tissue donor autograft. Gingival thickness is also required at the recipient site for techniques using a split-thickness, sandwich-type flap, or pouch and tunnel techniques.

Table 19.1 Treatment options for various clinical conditions

Existing Condition	Proposed Treatment
Lack of attached gingiva (≤ 1 mm) No recession Lack of vestibular depth	Free gingival autograft
Gingival recession (needed for root coverage) Miller's (1985) class I and II[a]	Connective tissue graft

	3.3- to 5.9-mm recessions
	   Average percentage of root coverage: 91%
	Coronally advanced flap
	   2.2- to 4.1-mm recession
	   Average percentage of root coverage: 83%
	Guided tissue regeneration
	   4.6- to 6.3-mm recession
	   Average percentage of root coverage: 74%
	Free gingival autograft
	   2.1- to 5.1-mm recessions
	   Average percentage of root coverage: 72%
	Rotational flaps
	   3- to 5-mm recession
	   Average percentage of root coverage: 64%
	Two-stage procedure
	   Average percentage of root coverage: 63%

Gingival recession Miller's (1985) class III and IV	Incomplete root coverage irrespective of the technique used
High insertion of labial maxillary or mandibular frenum, frenum pull, recession	Frenectomy for orthodontic treatment Frenectomy with or without free gingival autograft

Ridge deformities
Horizontal and vertical deficits, severe defects ≥ 4 mm[b]
	Fixed partial denture restoration planned
	   Soft tissue grafting (free gingival, connective tissue, Alloderm[c] grafts)
	Implant supported prosthesis planned
	   Hard tissue grafting (GBR, ERE)

Ridge deformities
Horizontal and vertical deficits, severe defects ≥ 4 mm[b]
	Fixed partial denture restoration planned
	   Soft tissue grafting (free gingival, connective tissue, AlloDerm[c] grafts)
	Implant-supported prosthesis planned
	   Hard tissue grafting (GBR), distraction osteogenesis
	Combination of soft and hard tissue grafting

Extensive caries, short clinical crowns, traumatic injuries, or severe parafunctional habits Compromised biological width High smile line showing excessive amounts of gingiva, resulting in patient's discontent with facial appearance Altered passive eruption	Crown-lengthening procedure with resective osseous surgery
Excessive gingival tissue covering erupted dentition (gingival hyperplasia, hypertrophy, pseudo-gingival pockets)	Soft tissue resective surgery (internal/external bevel gingivectomy, gingivoplasty)

[a] Adapted from Wennstrom (1996).
[b] Adapted from Pini-Prato et al. (2004).
[c] Acellular dermal matrix Allograft.
GBR, guided bone regeneration; ERE, edentulous ridge expansion.

GRAFT STABILITY

Good anastomosis of the blood vessels from the grafted donor tissue to the recipient site requires a stable environment. This necessitates sutures that stabilize the donor tissue firmly against the recipient site. The goal is maximum stability with the smallest number of sutures.

TRAUMA

Like all surgical procedures, periodontal plastic surgery is based on the meticulous, delicate, and precise management of the oral tissue. Unnecessary tissue trauma caused by poor incisions, flap perforations, tears, or traumatic and excessive placement of sutures can lead to tissue necrosis. The selection of proper instruments, needles, and sutures is necessary to minimize tissue trauma. The use of sharp, contoured blades, smaller-diameter needles, and resorbable, monofilament sutures is important in achieving atraumatic surgery (Table 19.1).

REFERENCES

Miller, P.D., Jr. (1985) A classification of marginal tissue recession. *International Journal of Periodontics and Restorative Dentistry* 5, 8–13.

Pini-Prato, G.P., Cairo, F., Tinti, C., Cortellini, P., Muzzi, L., & Mancini, E.A. (2004) Prevention of alveolar ridge deformities and reconstruction of lost anatomy: A review of surgical approaches. *International Journal of Periodontics and Restorative Dentistry* 24, 435–445.

Wennstrom, J.L. (1996) Mucogingival therapy. *Annals of Periodontology* 1, 671–701.

Index